PARIS VOGUE
COVERS

SONIA RACHLINE

PARIS VOGUE
COVERS

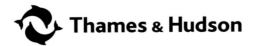
Thames & Hudson

Contents

Ninety years of *Vogue* covers

Mert Alas & Marcus Piggott
Richard Avedon
David Bailey
Eduardo Benito
Breitenmoser
Marc Chagall
René Chateau
Henry Clarke
G. Coltellacci
Salvador Dalí
Patrick Demarchelier
Robert Doisneau
Helen Dryden
Arthur Elgort
André François
Philippe Halsman
David Hockney
Horst P. Horst
George Hoyningen-Huene
Lionel Kazan
Tom Keogh

Bill King
Steven Klein
William Klein
Peter Knapp
Nick Knight
Akira Kurosawa
Inez van Lamsweerde
& Vinoodh Matadin
Georges Lepape
Peter Lindbergh
Craig McDean
Steven Meisel
Joan Miró
Jean-Baptiste Mondino
Tommy Mostwai
Pierre Mourgue
Arik Nepo
Nerebriarova
Helmut Newton
Terry O'Neill

Jean Pagès
Irving Penn
Georges W. Plank
Robert Randall
John Rawlings
Willy Rizzo
Pierre Roy
Richard Rutledge
Sempé
Jeanloup Sieff
David Sims
Mario Sorrenti
Edward Steichen
Bert Stern
Mario Testino
Sveeva Vigeveno
Andy Warhol
Albert Watson
Bruce Weber
Sabine Weiss
Alix Zeilinger

Foreword

Creating a cover is at once exciting and stressful. How can you be sure of your work – certain that you have got it right? And what is a good cover anyway? Is it one that encourages people to buy the magazine? Or where the quality of the image has lasting interest? One or two things you learn from experience: the visual immediacy of the graphics, a clearly defined goal, a model who looks straight at the camera and holds the reader's gaze, a touch of luxury – all of these work to one's advantage. Gold, silver, red and pink lettering work well, whereas green does not. Humour is appealing, nudity less so. And yet these guidelines alone are no guarantee of commercial or artistic success, as we see if we look back through the magazine's archives, trawling through ninety years of graphic design. This is particularly true of *Vogue*, which has traditionally relied on a bold, even iconoclastic approach. So, what does that mean? For a visually attuned person like myself, a good cover is a pleasure to look at, and has an impact that one can return to without getting tired of it, but it is also underpinned by an idea, a way of looking at things that is entirely subjective. At the end of the day, there is only one recipe for success as I see it: a cover must be true to itself.

Carine Roitfeld
Editor-in-Chief, *Paris Vogue*

VOGUE

Edition Française

15 Juin 1920

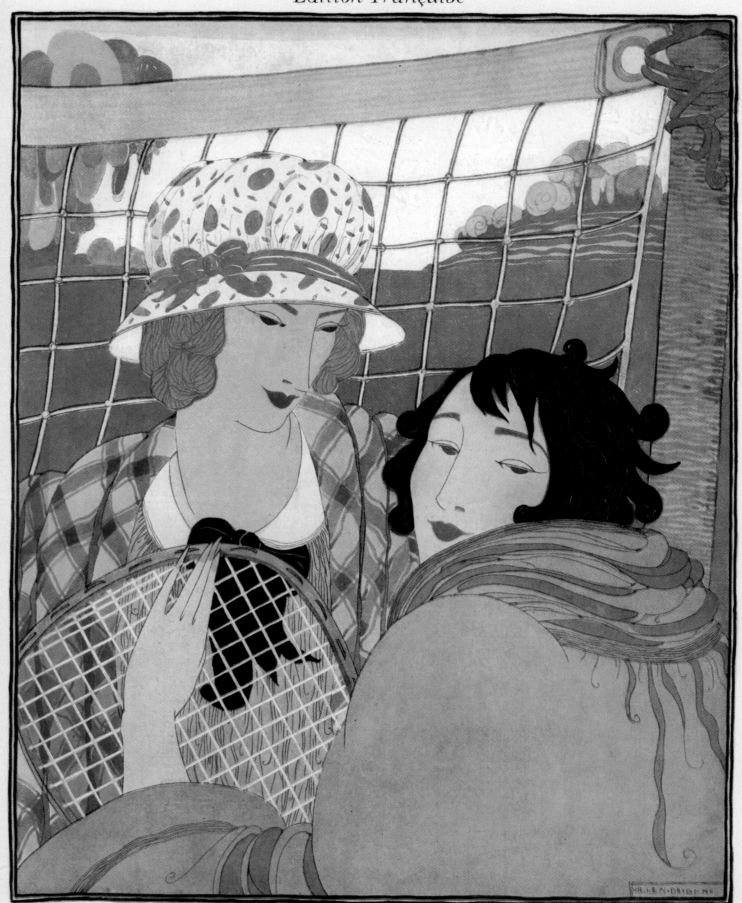

Editions Condé Nast

Prix 4 francs

Introduction

'Following her appearance on the cover of *Vogue*,
she moved effortlessly into café society – the self-regarding
group of artists, patrons and publishers.'
— Carolyn Burke, *Lee Miller: A Life*

The cover has a status distinct from the rest of a magazine. Unlike the other pages, it is seen as a collective work and not something that has been created by an illustrator alone, or a graphic designer, photographer, model, editor or other collaborator. Only the publication itself can claim ownership of, or rights to, this particular page. This is a legal point, but it also illustrates the specificity of the cover, which is simultaneously both a representation of the whole and a page of advertising, requiring sufficient character to communicate the spirit of the magazine and sufficient individuality to embody its difference.

This dual function as an informative document and a piece of marketing, moreover, reinforces its historical and socio-cultural interest: while reflecting a particular editorial stance, in order to be effective a cover must equally be of the moment. It must express a certain contemporaneity, the spirit and seductiveness of now, in order to win over its potential readers.

The covers of *Vogue*, and the selection offered here – images drawn from the ninety-year lifespan of the French edition – are in point of fact an ideal example:

11

not only do they offer a clear impression of the magazine's enduring artistic aspirations, they also enable us to survey a broad sweep of the history of style and elegance, of trends in fashion and aesthetics, of elitism too, all of which began in the early years of the 20th century and have left nothing to chance since then.

It all started in 1909, when Condé Nast, an American press and media aficionado, bought the then-failing magazine *Vogue*. Targeted at the upper-class women of New York, it was short on both funds and readers. Nast's development strategy for the magazine was to focus on a very specific area of the market rather than aiming for mass appeal. He wanted quality over quantity of readership, and he took it upon himself to address an elite and wealthy stratum of society who commanded the means to be seduced by upmarket advertising campaigns. His aim was to set higher advertising rates than those charged by the magazine's competitors on the grounds that *Vogue*'s readers were carefully targeted to be potential purchasers and trendsetters.

To explain what was a totally new concept, Nast invoked his now-famous metaphor: 'If you had a tray with two million needles on it and only one hundred and fifty thousand of these had gold tips, which you wanted, it would be an endless and costly process to weed them out. Moreover, the one million, eight hundred and fifty thousand which were not gold-tipped would be of no use to you, they couldn't help you; but if you could get a magnet that would draw only the gold ones, what a saving!'

Vogue was to become that magnet. Recognizing the powers of suggestion and seduction wielded by images and advertising, Condé Nast accorded primary importance to the cover, the fundamental point of contact with those he was seeking to reach. He also focused on fashion, since this was a matter of intimate concern to the elite – and the advertisers – in whom he was interested. He systematically enlisted the services of the finest illustrators and photographers, commissioning them to produce covers that were exquisitely judged and executed blends of art and chic, employing bold colours and striking graphics. In other words, he focused on the specific preferences of his target readers in order to capture their interest – a rule that he would apply equally fastidiously to the French edition of *Vogue*, which first came out in 1920.

Over the course of several decades, leading up to the Second World War, *Vogue* covers thus closely reflect the century's major artistic currents, no less than haute couture itself in its great hour of glory, or the style and lifestyle of the jet set; all of them were perfect icons of a society that was both restrained and extremely influential.

By the end of the 1940s, things were much changed. Shifting geographic frontiers, fluctuating hopes and fears for the future, and accelerating modernity all brought great uncertainty. *Vogue* and its covers were forced to evolve, but the magazine remained faithful nevertheless to its values and its aesthetic and artistic aspirations, which had more common ground with dreams than with everyday life. Everything had changed: the world that was being described, the tools used for describing it, and those to whom all this was being addressed. These changes had to be taken into account: the development, for example, of the consumer society and ready-to-wear in the 1950s, the emancipation of women in the 1960s, the sexual liberation of the 1970s, the emergence of international fashions in the 1980s, of the celebrity cult in the 1990s, and globalization at the start of the new millennium, as well as the ongoing evolution of the media and the luxury industries... The magazine honed its weapons in response, giving priority to committed photographers for whom the fashion photo was also and above all a means of personal expression, an opportunity to opt for the exception rather than the rule, and even sometimes an inclination to break the rules, to take a bold gamble on the future.

Back in the 1920s and 1930s, the artistic avant-garde were supported by the patronage of the French upper classes – Marie-Laure and Charles de Noailles being among the most famous of such patrons. Today, it is the big fashion groups who play that role, helping to bring such artists to the attention of a wider public. *Vogue* has enjoyed a privileged position throughout, as reflected by its covers, which in both conception and execution are in a class of their own. Carine Roitfeld, the magazine's Editor-in-Chief since 2001, puts it quite simply: 'What is ordinary for us is ... extraordinary.'

Famous illustrations

'Class, not mass'
— Condé Nast

During the 1920s and 1930s, the logistics of taking a fashion photograph were such that it was difficult to produce more than ten shots a month. Was this the reason why the covers of that period relied by far the most frequently on illustrations?

It is a tempting explanation, and yet it cannot account for the artistic quality of the cover designs published by *Vogue* at that time, and it was itself, rather, the fruit of an encounter between the bigger and the smaller picture, between the Paris of the *Années Folles* – the Roaring Twenties – and the magazine.

At the start of the 20th century, two cultural events exercised a profound influence on Paris life, contributing, in passing, to the demise of Art Nouveau: on the one hand, there was Sergei Diaghilev's Ballets Russes, which burst on to the stage of the Théâtre du Châtelet in 1909 and provided a revolutionary aesthetic experience combining dance, music, poetry and painting, against a flamboyantly exotic background, and over the years involved the collaboration of Picasso, Matisse, Braque, Cocteau, Mallarmé, Ravel and Debussy. The other event was the opening of a *maison de couture* by the enlightened and insatiably curious Paul Poiret, a man who was drawn to all things modern and took his inspiration from every contemporary trend – from Fauvism to Constructivism via the Ballets Russes, of which he was a fervent admirer. From the outset, Poiret raised fashion to the status of an artistic creation in its own right, freeing the feminine form from the physical and social prison of the corset, experimenting with a painter's palette and creating Oriental-style lines that were totally new in terms both of comfort and daring. With Poiret, clothing and art discovered common ground, clearly and directly linked in a way that had never been seen before. Poiret commissioned fabric designs from Raoul Dufy and employed leading illustrators to depict his models. Paul Iribe and Georges Lepape designed his brochures in 1908 and 1911 respectively.

For the first time ever, artists, designers and couturiers started to frequent the same theatrical events and private views and dinner parties, forming a small circle of aesthetes dedicated to challenging traditional cultural values. One of their number, Lucien Vogel, another arbiter of taste, played a prominent part in strengthening and formalizing these links. Vogel was a publisher and artistic director of considerable talent. The son of an illustrator, he was married to Cosette de Brunhoff (sister of Jean de Brunhoff, creator of Babar the Elephant) and had worked alongside his father-in-law on the production of the Ballets Russes catalogues. He was very much in tune with his times and in 1912 launched the *Gazette du bon ton*, an art and fashion magazine in which his painter and illustrator friends reproduced and interpreted models by the great couturiers such as Cherwit, Doeuillet, Doucet, Paquin, Poiret, Redfern and Worth. The *Gazette* thus became a showpiece for the likes of André Marty, Pierre Mourgue, Georges Lepape, Léon Bakst, George Barbier and Pierre Brissaud, among others, while members of the aristocracy and the *grande bourgeoisie* formed a loyal readership.

Given Vogel's credentials, it is no surprise that Condé Nast should have chosen to enlist his services for the French edition of the magazine, which he launched to join the American and English editions in 1920. Since buying *Vogue* in 1909, Nast had continued to pursue the editorial strategies that he had established from the start, aiming his magazine squarely at an international elite which had a taste for, and the means to purchase, those – essentially fashion – goods displayed in the pages of *Vogue* through advertising inserts sold to the luxury labels at higher rates than anywhere else. Condé Nast knew that the general quality of the magazine and its covers in particular were crucial if it was to attract the right readership: this elite group of readers needed to recognize themselves in the magazine at a glance.

Lucien Vogel was clearly the man for the job, the perfect point of contact between the worlds of publishing, fashion and art, the privileged middleman whose instincts were as sound as his address book. Condé Nast had known him since 1915, when he had proposed the idea of co-publishing a special issue of the *Gazette du bon ton* to coincide with the Universal Exposition held in San Francisco. Thus he offered Vogel the job of Art Director on *Vogue*, appointed his wife Cosette as Editor, and acquired the *Gazette du bon ton* in the process.

This was 1920, the perfect moment for launching the magazine: the First World War may have rudely interrupted the jubilant rhythm of Paris life, but since 1918 this had resumed with even greater brio. The 1920s were from the outset a time of continuous celebration in the capital – a time of partying, pleasure, culture and escapism, in which the assurance of victory mingled with the desire to forget as speedily as possible the massive privations and losses inflicted by the war. This made Paris a magnet for a host of international interests and talents.

The atmosphere encouraged people to spend money, to enjoy themselves and to break free from the past: advertising was booming; couturiers were bursting with inspiration; and avant-garde trends – which reached their highpoint with the Exposition des Arts Décoratifs in 1925 – helped to de-sanctify art, obliterating the boundaries between fine and applied arts, and creating a surge of artists eager to put their inspiration in the service of more commercial projects.

It was in Paris, therefore, that everything was happening. Condé Nast understood this perfectly, and Edna Woolman Chase, American *Vogue*'s legendary Editor (who was to hold the reins up until 1952), travelled to Paris as often as she was able. In fact, although a great many of the magazine's pages were common to all three editions, it was most often from Paris, rather than New York or London, that their creative energy and glamour emanated during those years.

French *Vogue* was in a very strong position, supported on the one hand by its American-style marketing strategy and on the other by the existence of its local dream team (Lucien and Cosette Vogel were soon to be joined by another Brunhoff sibling, Michel, also a talented aficionado of the arts), and was thus able to achieve a perfect balance between the people who created the magazine, the people who appeared in its pages and the people who read it. Nothing could have been neater: the upper classes – the Noailles among them – patronized the artists; the artists collaborated with the top couturiers; the couturiers dressed the upper classes and invested in advertising; advertisements, consisting of illustrations by the artists, appeared in *Vogue*; and *Vogue* reflected the aristocratic glamour that essentially interested … the aristocracy itself, the couturiers and the artists.

Vogue covers from the 1920s and 1930s bear the signature of many illustrious names, such as Eduardo Benito, Georges Lepape, Georges W. Plank, Éric, Helen Dryden, Jean Pagès, Giulio Coltellacci, Pierre Mourgue, Alix Zeilinger and Christian Bérard, and they illustrate this perfect complicity: for the most part, they carry little or no text, since the illustrator's style was sufficient identification in itself. There might be little fashion detail either: the intention was to reflect an attitude, a state of mind, an aesthetic stance first and foremost. The cover was an emblem of high society.

These covers are important art-historical documents: their images and logos were produced by genuine artists and developed out of the aesthetic movements of the time. Their coloured line drawings, many of them stencilled, reflect the Orientalist influence of the Ballets Russes and the gathering momentum of Art Deco, Cubist geometries and Surrealism. As such, they form a legitimate part of our international cultural heritage.

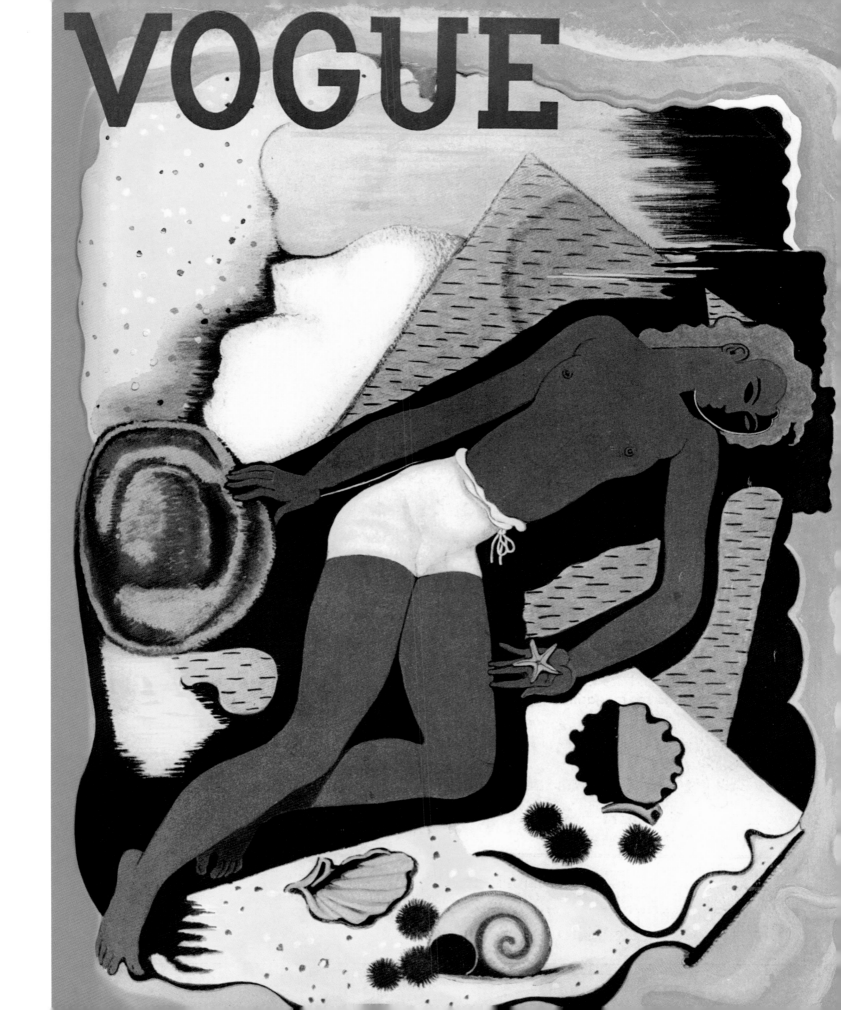

VOGUE

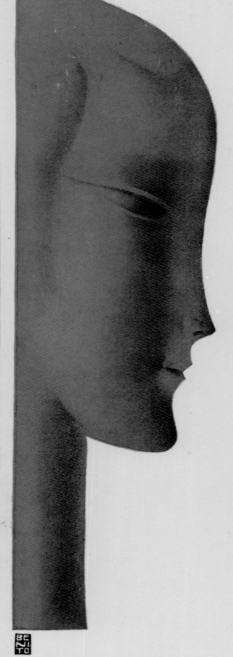

BE
NI
TO

PRÉVISIONS SUR
LA MODE DE PRINTEMPS

FÉVRIER 1929
PRIX 6 FRANCS

REVUE MENSUELLE
LES ÉDITIONS CONDÉ NAST

VOGUE

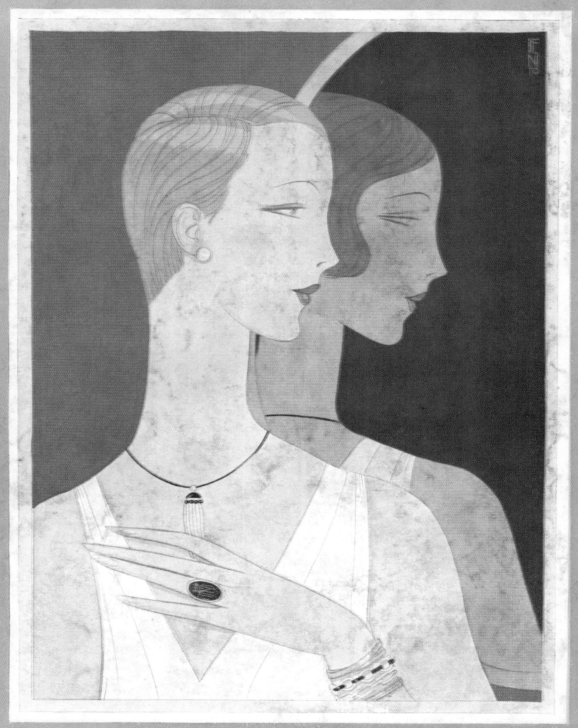

Les Nouvelles Collections
de
Printemps

1er Avril 1926   Revue Mensuelle   Prix 5 francs
LES ÉDITIONS CONDÉ NAST

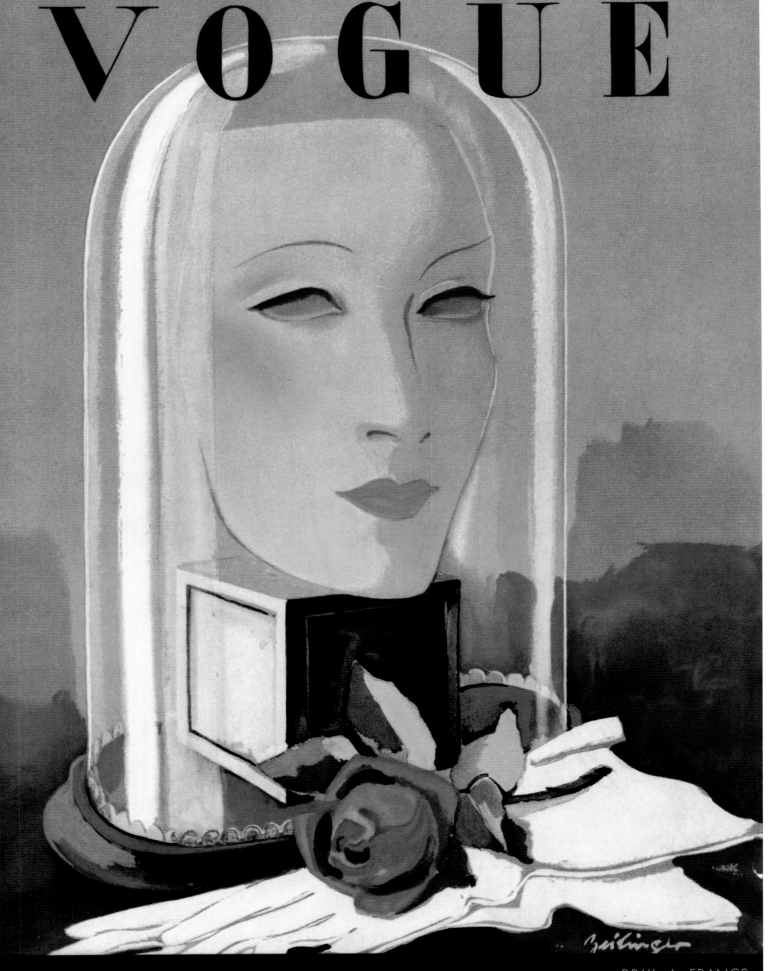

VOGUE

JANVIER 1935   LA LINGERIE   LES CROISIERES   PRIX 6 FRANCS

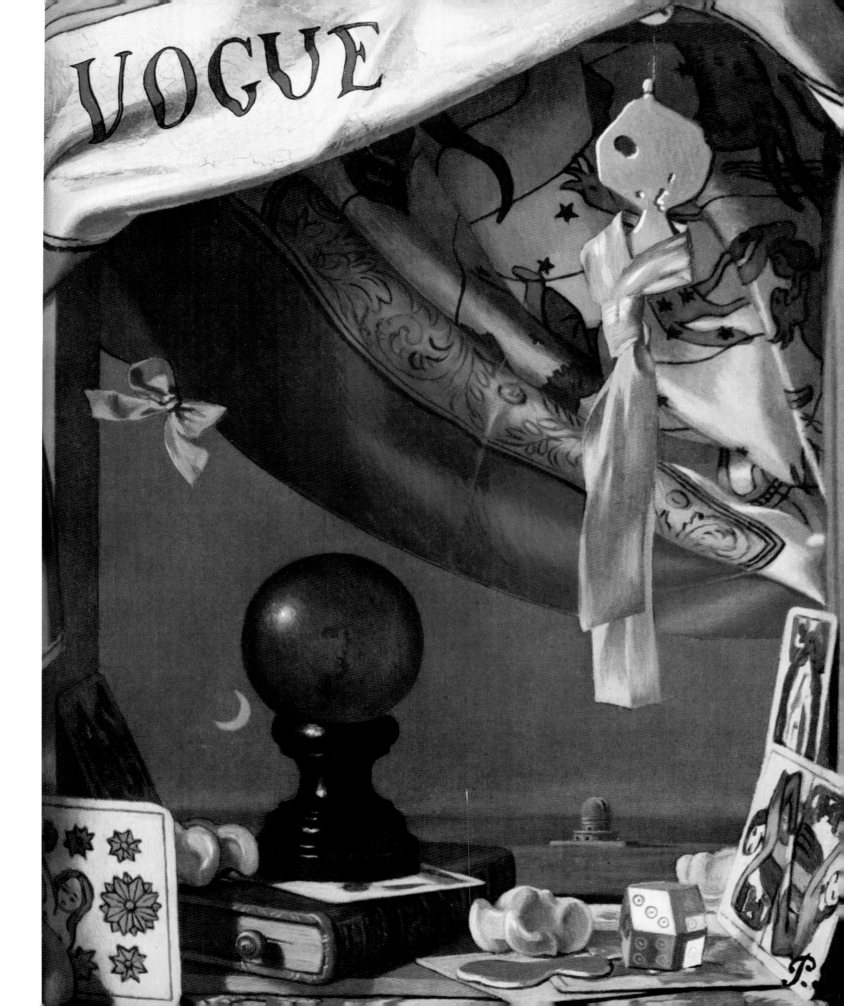

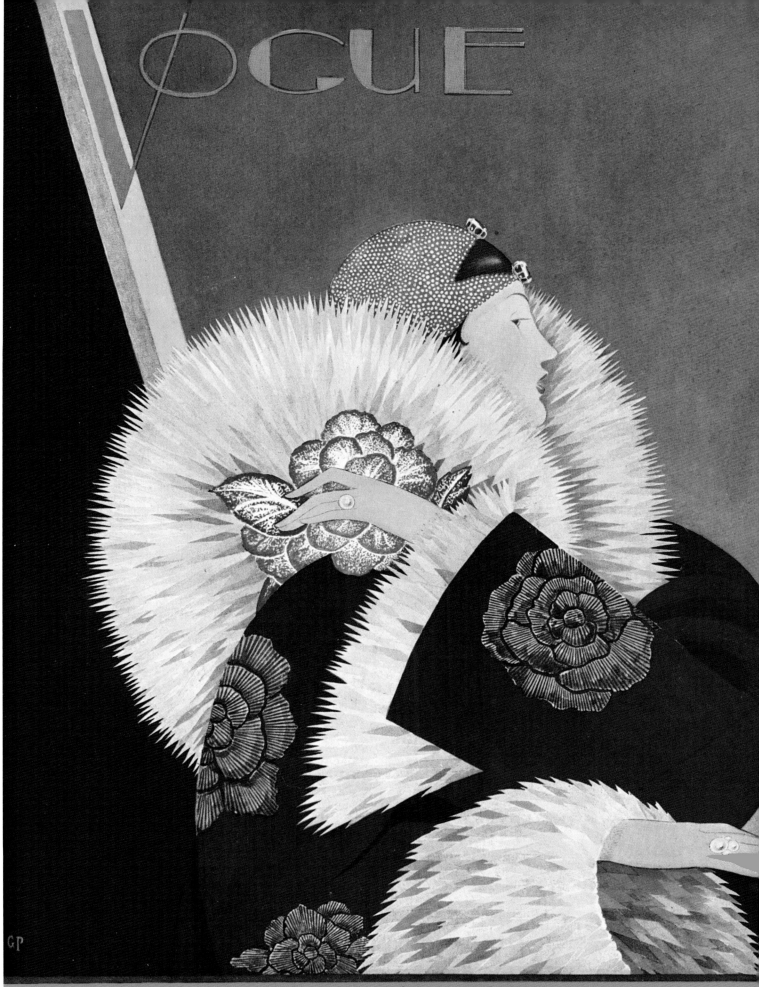

VOGUE

Prédictions sur les Modes de Printemps

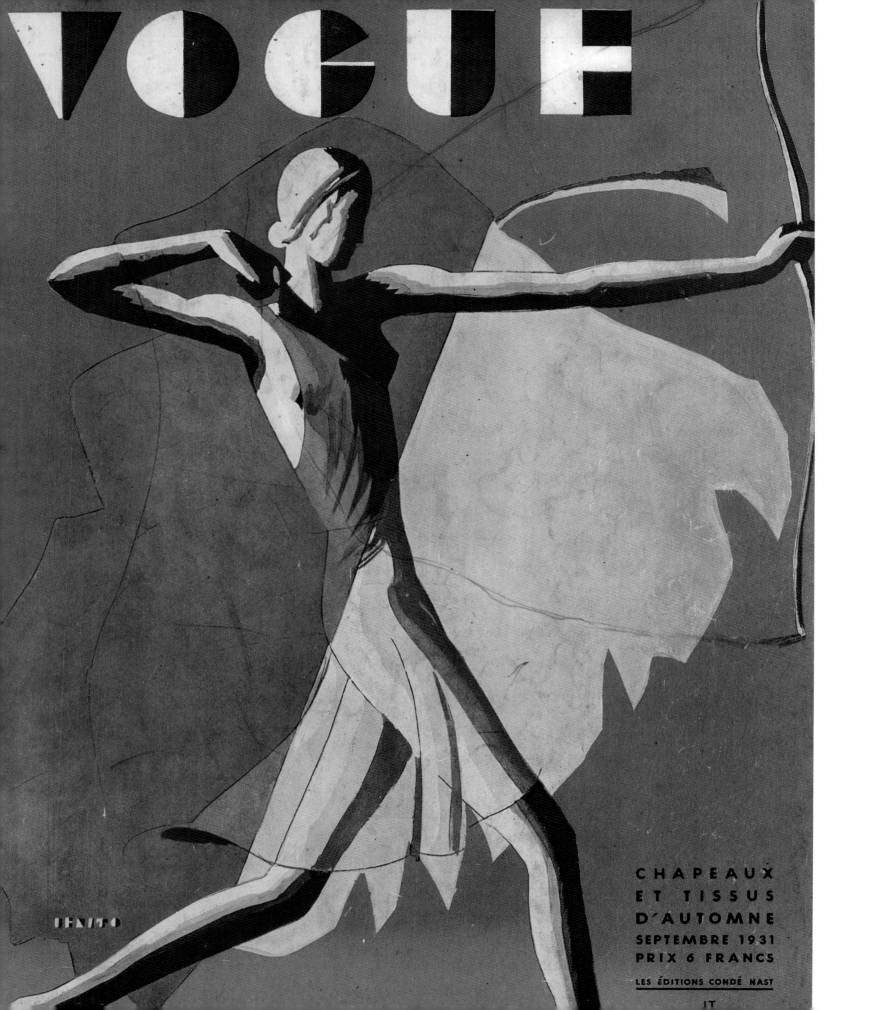

VOGUE

BENITO

CHAPEAUX
ET TISSUS
D'AUTOMNE
SEPTEMBRE 1931
PRIX 6 FRANCS

LES ÉDITIONS CONDÉ NAST

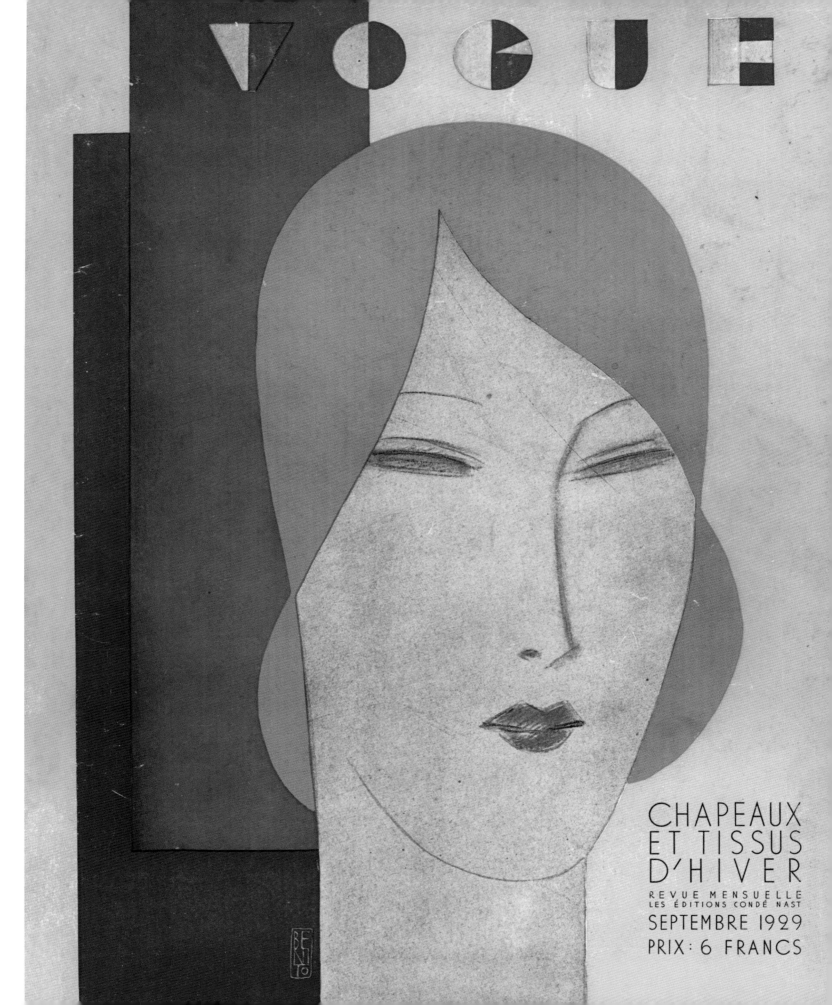

VOGUE

CHAPEAUX
ET TISSUS
D'HIVER
REVUE MENSUELLE
LES ÉDITIONS CONDÉ NAST
SEPTEMBRE 1929
PRIX: 6 FRANCS

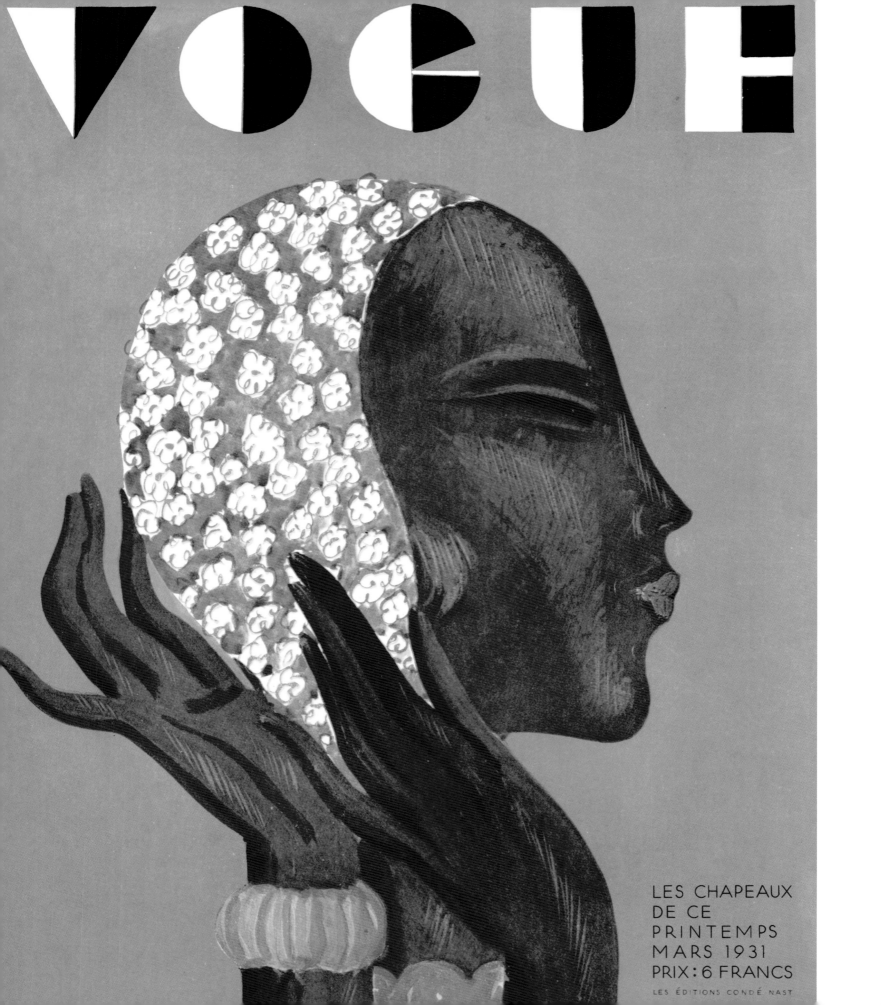

VOGUE

LES CHAPEAUX
DE CE
PRINTEMPS
MARS 1931
PRIX : 6 FRANCS

LES ÉDITIONS CONDÉ NAST

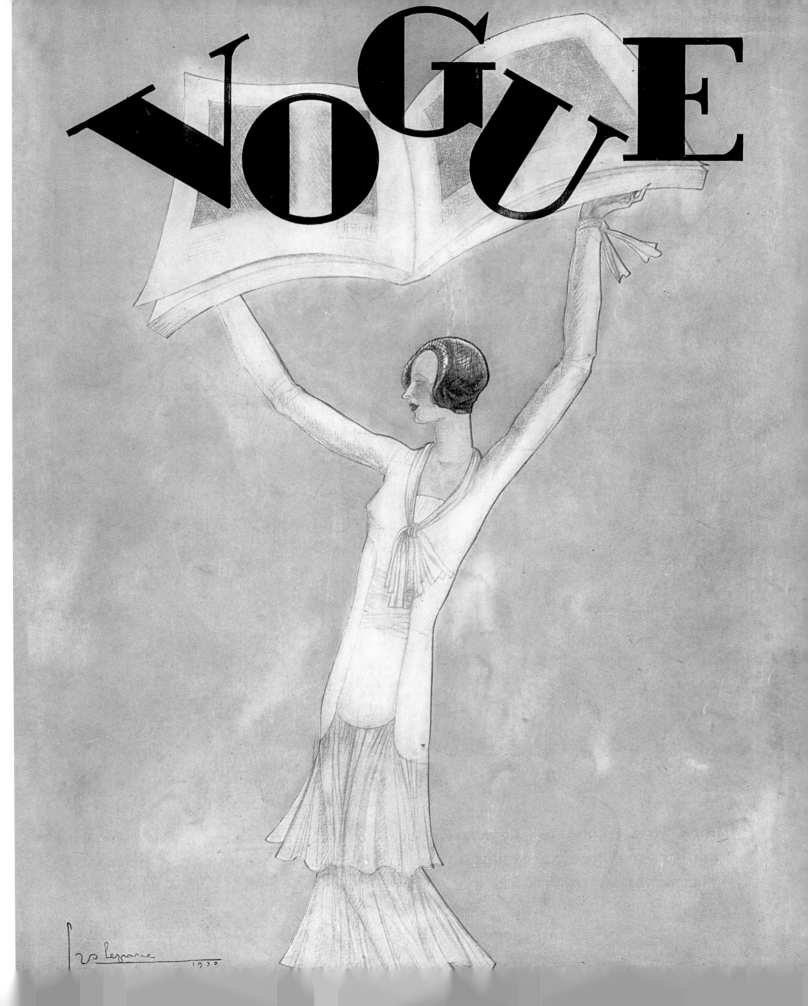

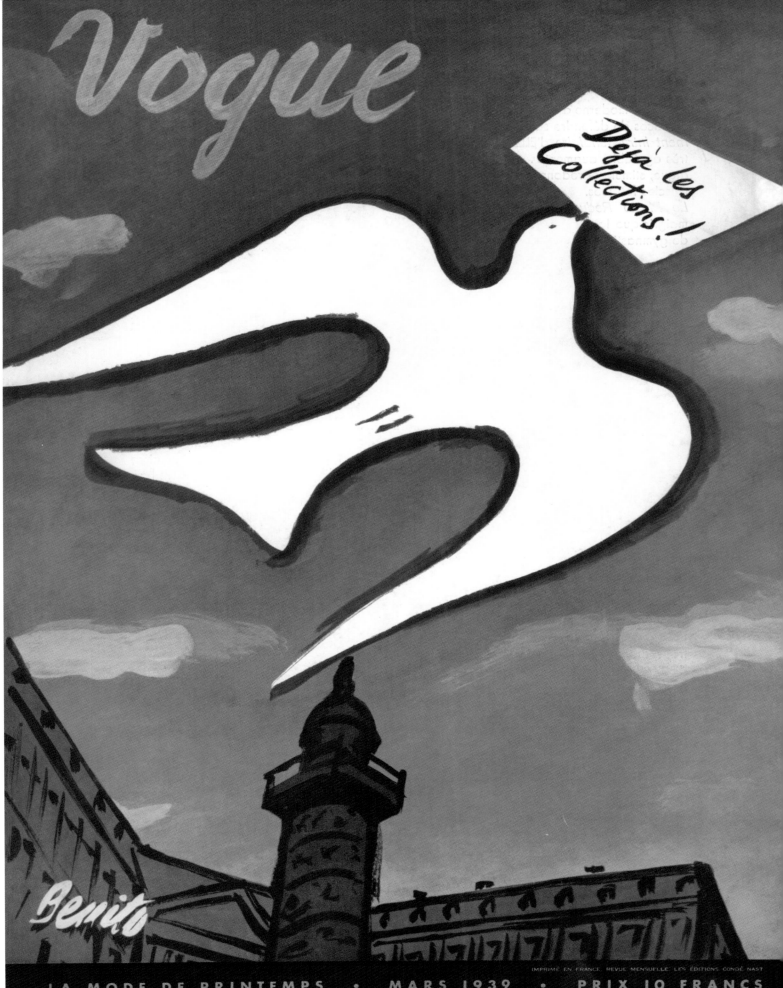

The studio, theatre of fashion

'Fashion can be bought. Style one must possess.'
— Edna Woolman Chase

Vogue covers began to display photographs from the early 1930s. They were signed by Edward Steichen, George Hoyningen-Huene and Horst P. Horst and were taken more often than not in the *Vogue* studio.

Steichen was a close friend of Picasso, Matisse and Brancusi, and was Condé Nast's chief photographer from 1923. A renowned and wealthy artist, resident in New York, he was known for his portraits of the stars and admired for his modernity – in other words, his willingness (and ability) to place his art in the service of advertising and the press. Baron George Hoyningen-Huene fled Russia in the company of his parents at the start of the 1917 Revolution. A precociously talented photographer and a great admirer of Steichen, he was appointed chief photographer at French *Vogue* in the mid-1920s, and it was there that, in 1930, he met Horst, a young German art student who became his assistant, his model and his lover prior to turning to photography himself. The model and future photographer Lee Miller was also doing her apprenticeship at the *Vogue* studios, in the Avenue des Champs-Élysées, at the time. Her biographer

Carolyn Burke describes what it was like: 'Their workplace resembled a stage set. Models posed on platforms lit by brilliant lights that threatened to melt their makeup. Assistants wheeled the large studio cameras into position, raised and lowered them on their wooden frames, then turned a wheel to move the lens in or out.'[1]

The fact that the magazine's fashion photos, and in particular those destined for the cover, were conceived indoors in the studio was in part a necessary consequence of complicated logistics. A range of factors, including the complex manipulations of the cameras, the very delicate colouring processes, décors requiring sometimes as long as a week to assemble, and the fact that the basic materials – photographic paper, developing chemicals, etc. – had to be imported from the United States, meant that only about ten photographs could be produced each month, some of them destined also to appear in the American and English editions of the magazine.

Quite aside from these constraints, however, the studio was like a stage, complete with sets and metamorphoses, and as such was the ideal vehicle for communicating the image of femininity as encapsulated by *Vogue*. It reflected an aesthetic perfectly suited to the Hollywood diva-style glamour of the 1930s: a type of beauty-on-a-pedestal that was at the heart of the couture ideal of the time, and whose focus was resolutely closer to the world of art than to everyday life.

A great many artists who were friends of the photographers hung around behind the scenes. Simone Eyrard, who came to work for the magazine as a retoucher in 1933 (and only left 47 years later), describes the atmosphere of tangible excitement that prevailed at the time of the collections: 'The cyclists fetched the dresses from the couturiers. That was usually in the evening, once the fashion parades were over. Then the models were closeted away for the photos. The Duchesse d'Ayen, who was the Fashion Editor, took care of their hair and their makeup herself... Once the session was finished, the cyclists rushed off again to return the dresses, while we started the developing. It took a fair bit of time, so we would go and see a review at Le Tabarin while we waited... Then we'd retrieve the contacts and dash to the Vert Galant, where Horst and Huene, surrounded by all their pals – Cocteau, Jean Marais, Boris Kochno, Christian Bérard, etc. – were waiting for us so that they could make their selection. After that, we'd go back to the lab for the printing and retouching, which we did with a scraper. We'd be up all night, and next morning everything was ready...'[2]

The offices of *Vogue France* were closed during the war and the Occupation, but when publication resumed in 1947 the studio began operating with increased vitality. Techniques were becoming simpler, and now that the photographers were back in Paris, more of them than ever gravitated towards the magazine. Some were commissioned by American *Vogue*, others by the French office, and they included Irving Penn, Cecil Beaton, Richard Rutledge, Arik Nepo, William Klein, Henry Clarke, Guy Bourdin, Helmut Newton and David Bailey, among others. There were two talent spotters, each with a keen eye and his own particular sensibilities: Alex Liberman, Art Director and later Editorial Director of Condé Nast Publications (a post he held up until the age of 82, in 1994), who was quick to pick out Penn and Klein; and Michel de Brunhoff, Editor of French *Vogue* (1929–54), who discovered and encouraged Guy Bourdin, among others. Yves Saint Laurent recalled his perceptiveness in an interview with Susan Train: 'Before I went to Dior's, Michel had got me to draw some hairstyles for *Vogue*. I was at their offices. There was a boy of about my age in a corner and Michel said to me, "See that young man? He's going to be a very great photographer." It was Bourdin! Michel had particularly sensitive antennae…'[3]

The American and the French editions had a successful working relationship: while the seasonal collections were being shown, the Americans produced most of their fashion series in Paris, and because they had a much bigger picture budget than the French office, they shared their photographs with them. By common agreement, the photos were attributed to one or other of the two magazines. And even though American *Vogue* offered more attractive rates, the top photographers were still keen to work for the French edition, which allowed them greater freedom of style and mood than any other magazine. There were no constraints – other than the obligation to exercise their creativity – and the magazine provided the ideal springboard for a photographer who wanted to get his work known and show off a distinctive style. The covers themselves were a direct expression of these creative aspirations: whereas American *Vogue* favoured a strategy of accessibility and complicity – faces in close-up, their eyes fixed on the potential purchaser, along with a choice of realistically wearable clothes – the covers of French *Vogue* were as eclectic as their photographers. For the most part, the model would be looking towards the camera, but otherwise they appeared to eschew any resolutely commercial logic. Straplines continued to be succinct and, as on the illustrated covers of the pre-war period, fashion per se and the promotion of a particular name were not systematic priorities, other than in exceptional cases such as Courrèges' futurist white, where the creator adopted a particularly bold stance.

Generally speaking, *Vogue* covers have always set out to define an attitude and a femininity that were specific to the magazine. In the 1930s this was expressed as a diva-style glamour and some thirty years later by adherence to a certain modernity. This change of style was clearly a matter of context: the 1950s and 1960s witnessed the emergence of a new phenomenon – ready-to-wear – which rapidly began to dominate the fashion scene. For *Vogue*, the magazine of the top couturiers, this revolutionary turning point was not always self-evident. Susan Train recalls a conversation that took place between Michel de Brunhoff and Edna Woolman Chase in 1952: 'Edna looked at Michel and said, "You know, of course, that the future of *Vogue France* depends on ready-to-wear." Michel went red, then white, then green, becoming almost hysterical. "But we'll lose all our advertisers," he exploded. To which Edna replied: "Trust me."'

The magazine came under pressure from a number of couturiers, including Balenciaga – who actually threatened to boycott it – but Michel de Brunhoff took the risk of believing Edna Woolman Chase. Ready-to-wear appeared in *Vogue*. But because its editors had every intention of remaining faithful to their readers and to the spirit of *Vogue* – that quintessential aestheticism and elitist chic without which the magazine was unthinkable – its covers gambled now on cutting-edge designs that were often non-conformist and sometimes avant-garde. These striking images continued to highlight its distinctive character, combining wearability with chic elegance and reserve in photographs that were sometimes extremely posed... It therefore continued to be easier to produce the photographs for these highly graphic, supremely modern covers in the studio rather than in an external setting. For practical reasons – limited space, fashion stories and teams that were becoming increasingly international – the Paris *Vogue* studio closed for good in 1994. But while over the years photographers have sought to work more and more in natural light, and in natural surroundings, the studio remains the ultimate theatrical setting, the ideal stage for the deployment of art, fashion, femininity and allure.

1 *Lee Miller: A Life*, Knopf, New York, 2005.

2 Interview conducted in 1995 by Susan Train, Paris Editor for American *Vogue* from 1951 to 1985; she later took charge of the Paris office of Condé Nast Publications, Inc.

3 Interview conducted in 1995.

May 1939
Horst P. Horst

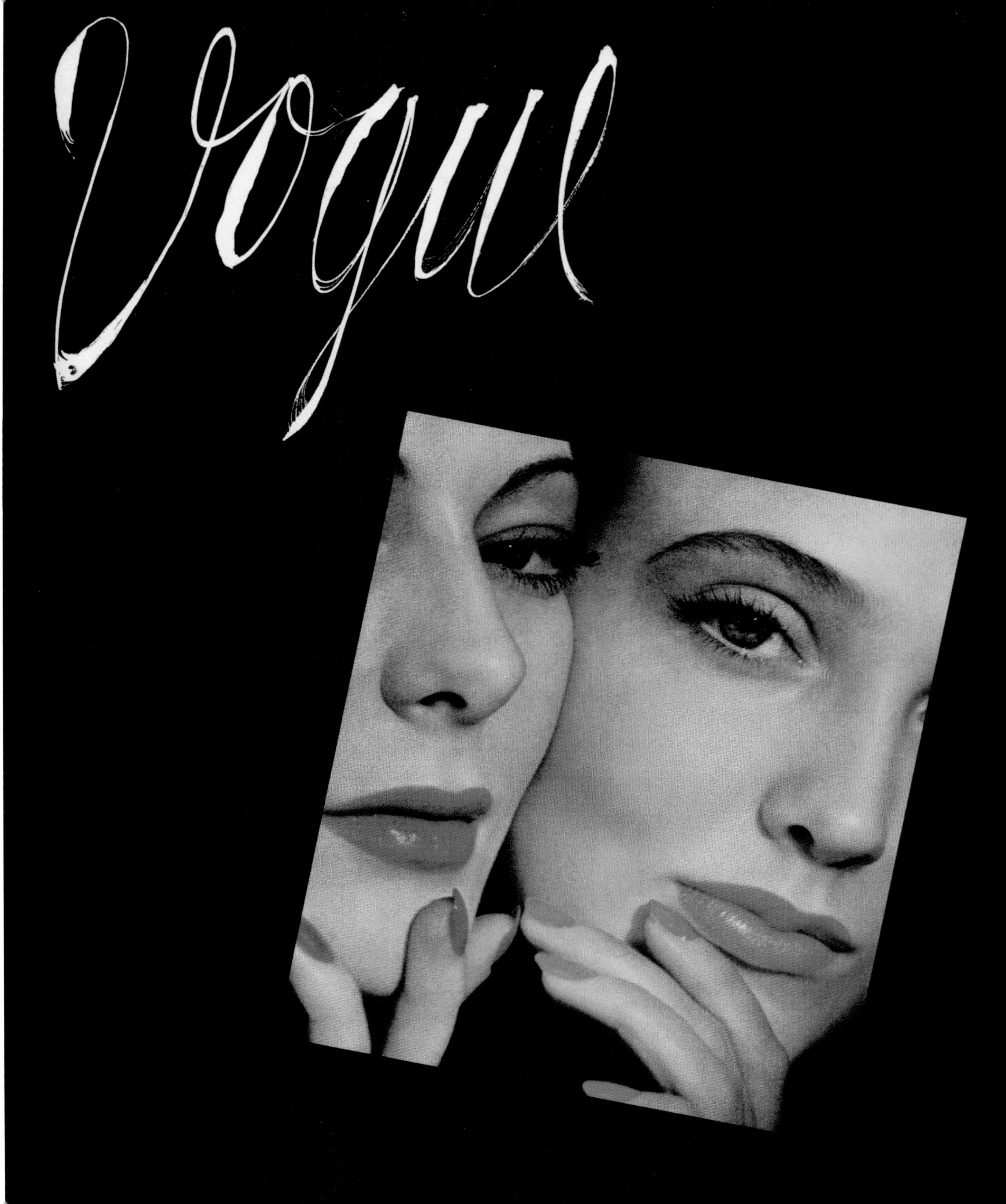
Vogue

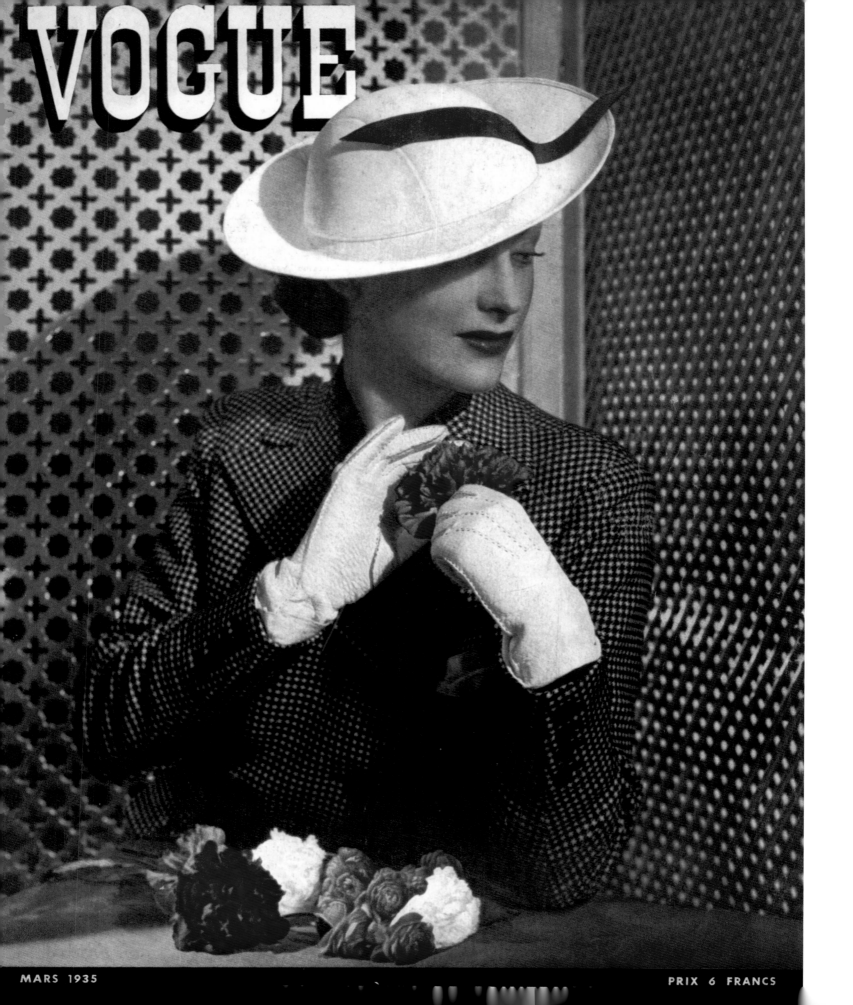

VOGUE

MARS 1935

PRIX 6 FRANCS

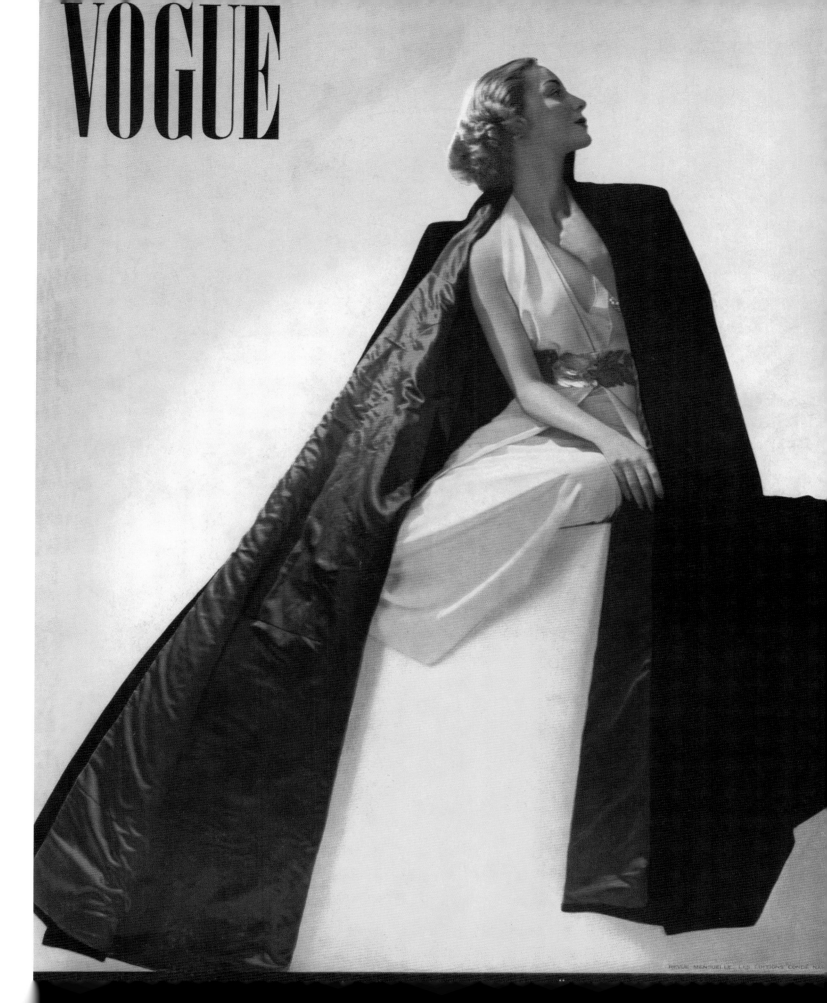

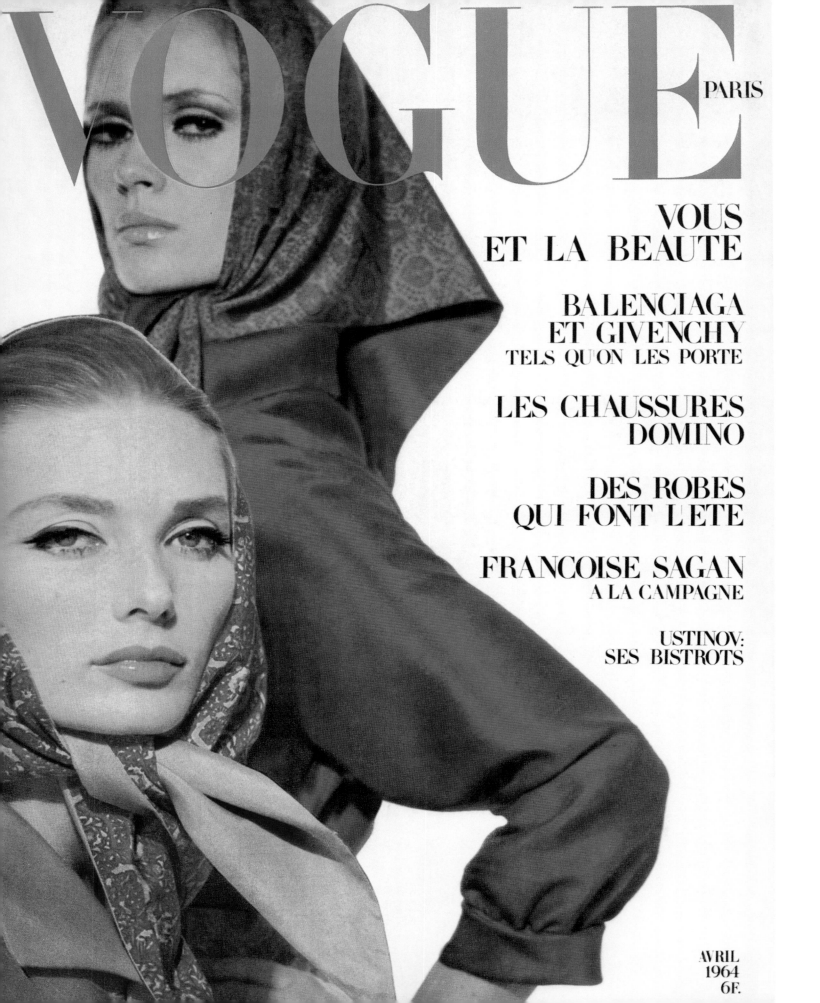

VOGUE PARIS

VOUS
ET LA BEAUTE

BALENCIAGA
ET GIVENCHY
TELS QU'ON LES PORTE

LES CHAUSSURES
DOMINO

DES ROBES
QUI FONT L'ETE

FRANCOISE SAGAN
A LA CAMPAGNE

USTINOV:
SES BISTROTS

AVRIL
1964
6F.

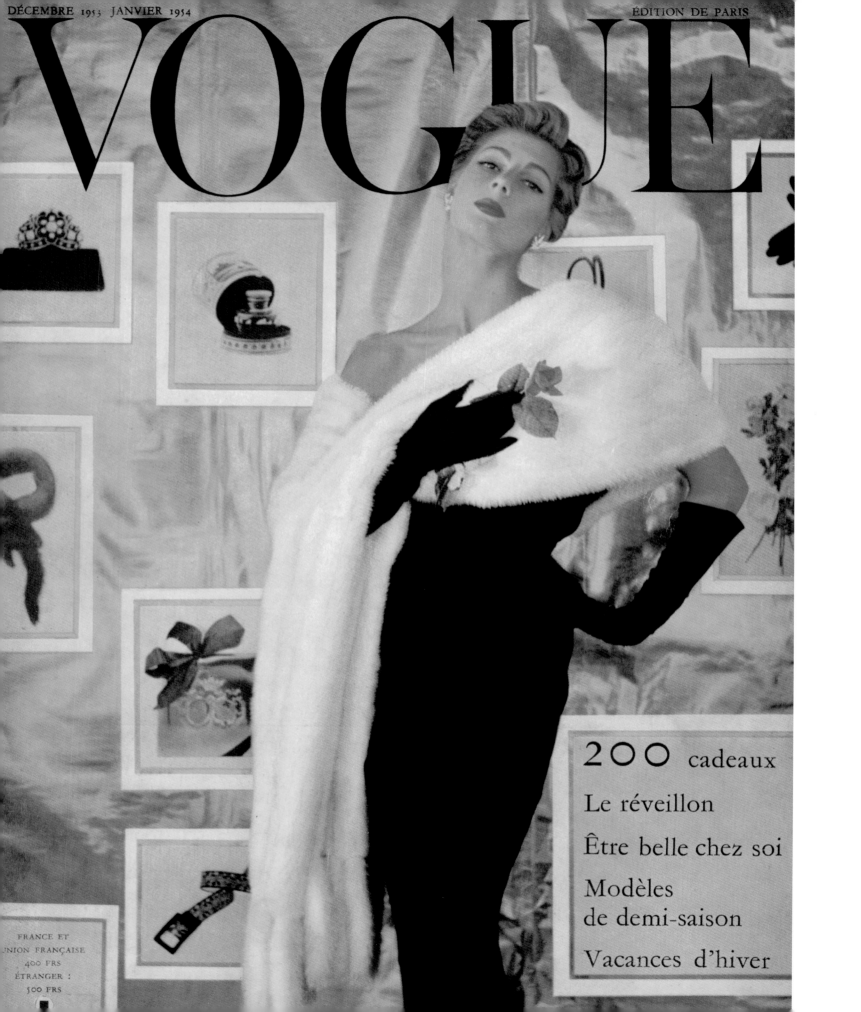

DÉCEMBRE 1953 JANVIER 1954

ÉDITION DE PARIS

VOGUE

200 cadeaux

Le réveillon

Être belle chez soi

Modèles
de demi-saison

Vacances d'hiver

FRANCE ET
UNION FRANÇAISE
400 FRS

ÉTRANGER :
500 FRS

VOGUE

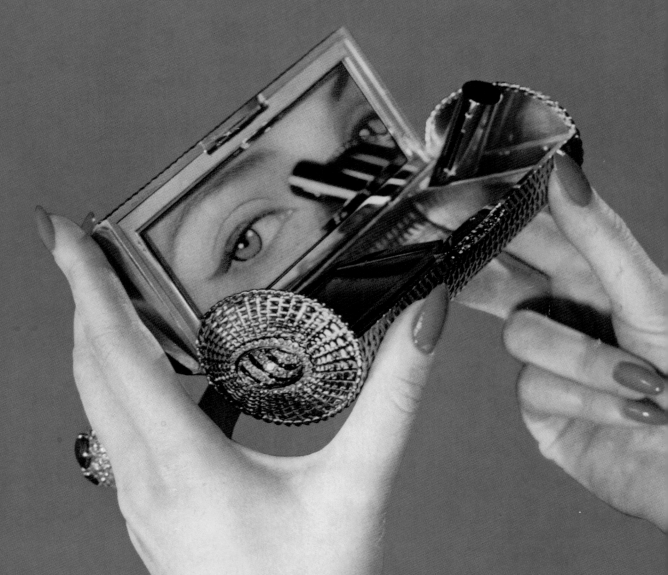

LA VIE A PARIS

**LES COLLECTIONS DE
DEMI-SAISON**

LE SKI - LES CADEAUX

DÉCEMBRE 1950 · JANVIER 1951 · REVUE MENSUELLE · IMPRIMÉE EN FRANCE · PRIX : 500 FR

PREVIOUS PAGES
December 1953
Sabine Weiss

December 1950
Arik Nepo

OPPOSITE
October 1950
Irving Penn

VOGUE

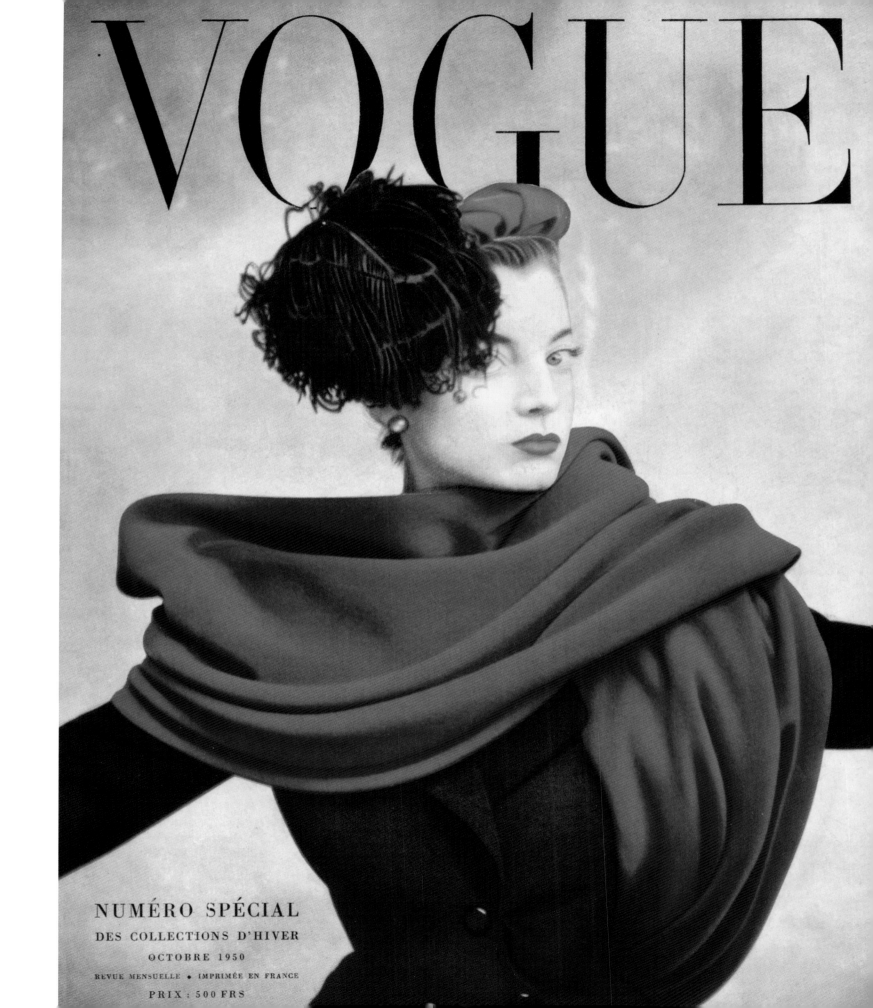

NUMÉRO SPÉCIAL

DES COLLECTIONS D'HIVER

OCTOBRE 1950

REVUE MENSUELLE · IMPRIMÉE EN FRANCE

PRIX : 500 FRS

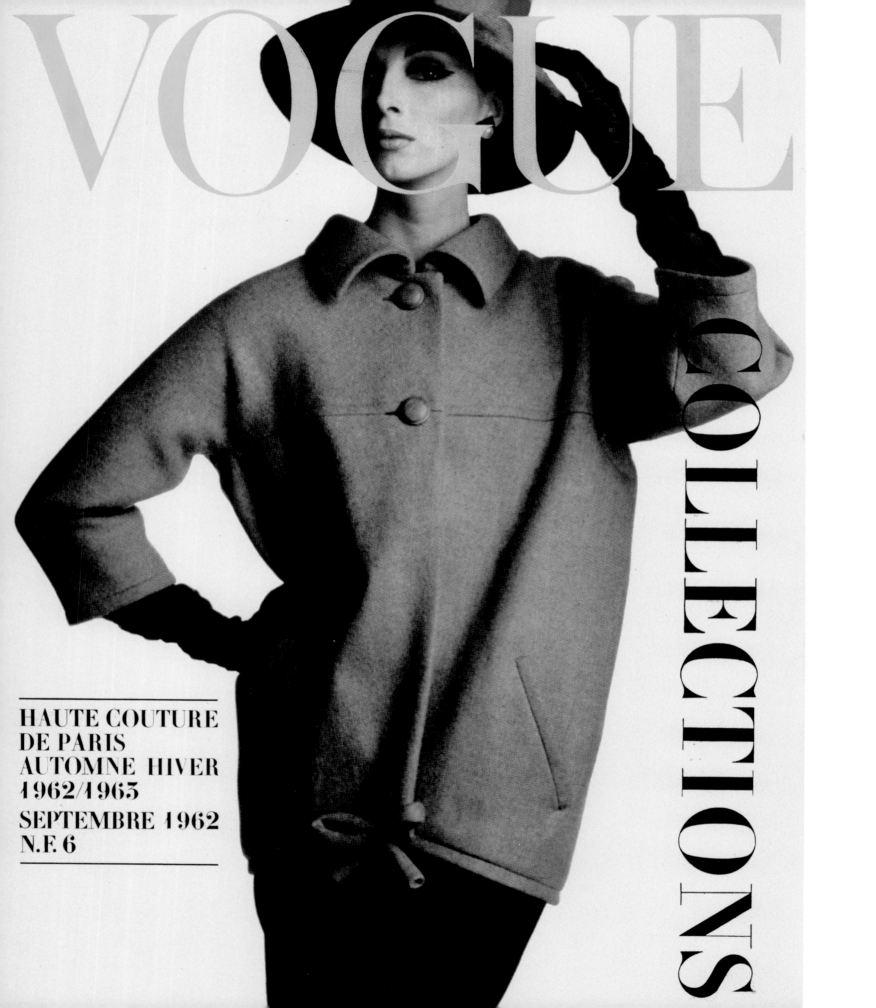

VOGUE

COLLECTIONS

HAUTE COUTURE
DE PARIS
AUTOMNE HIVER
1962/1963
SEPTEMBRE 1962
N.F. 6

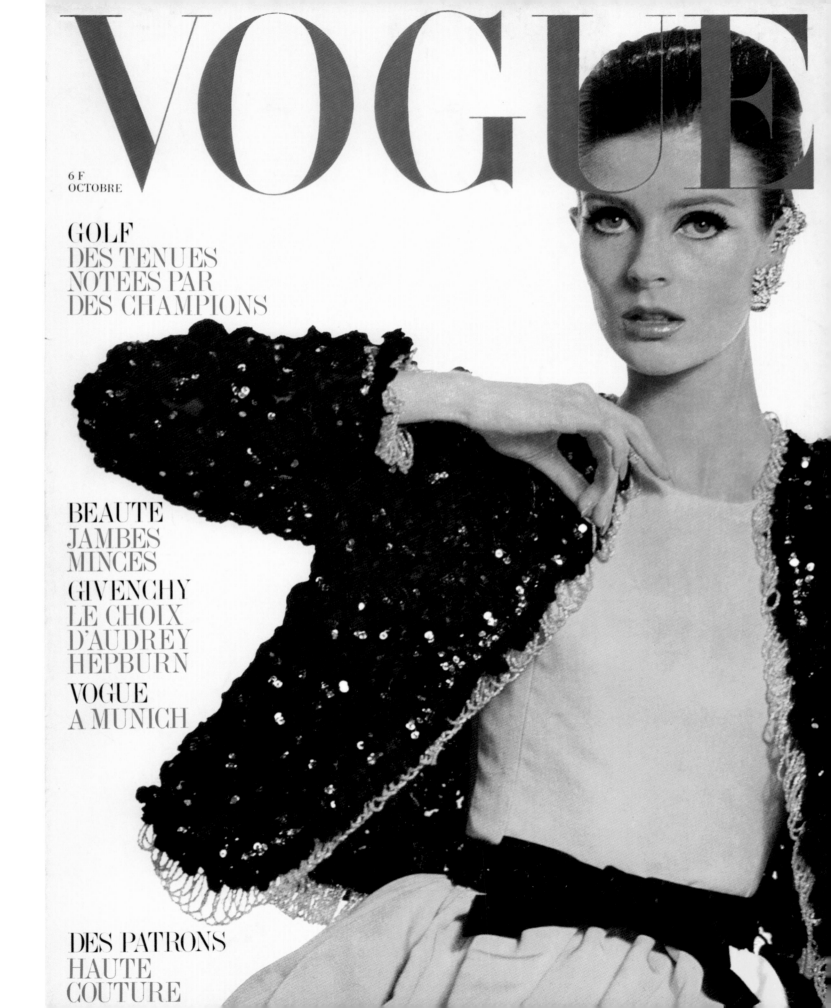

VOGUE

6 F
OCTOBRE

GOLF
DES TENUES
NOTÉES PAR
DES CHAMPIONS

BEAUTÉ
JAMBES
MINCES

GIVENCHY
LE CHOIX
D'AUDREY
HEPBURN

VOGUE
A MUNICH

DES PATRONS
HAUTE
COUTURE

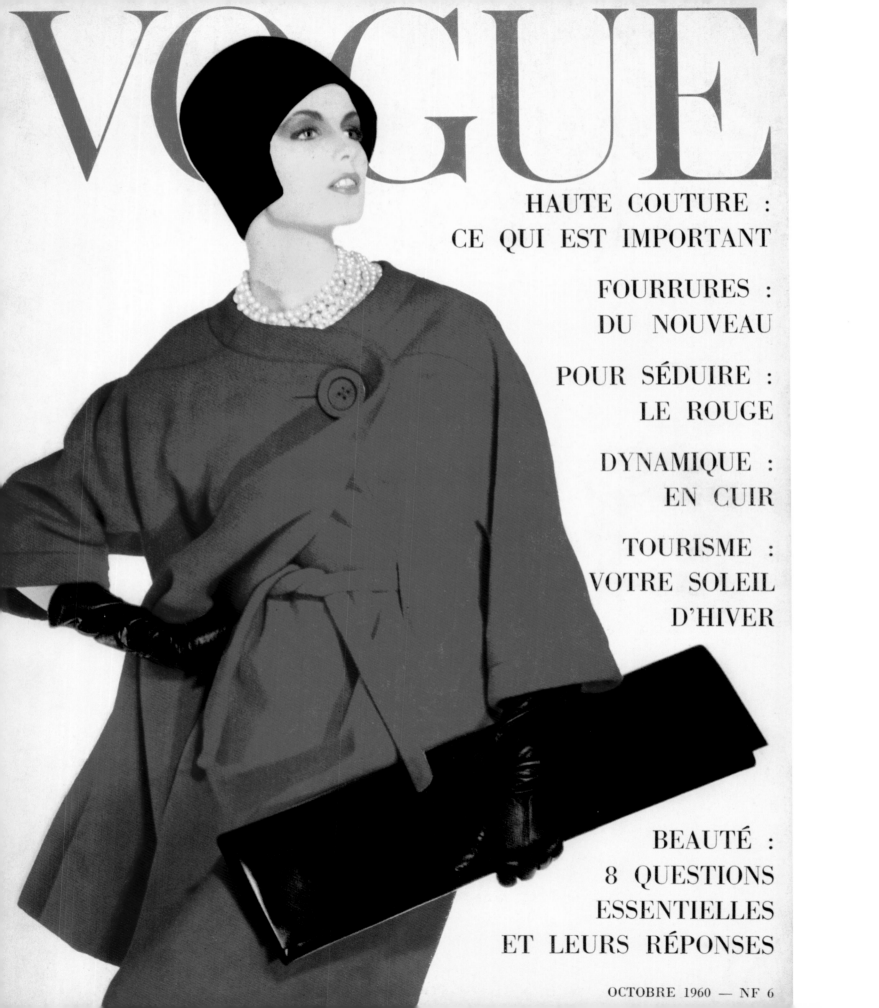

VOGUE

HAUTE COUTURE :
CE QUI EST IMPORTANT

FOURRURES :
DU NOUVEAU

POUR SÉDUIRE :
LE ROUGE

DYNAMIQUE :
EN CUIR

TOURISME :
VOTRE SOLEIL
D'HIVER

BEAUTÉ :
8 QUESTIONS
ESSENTIELLES
ET LEURS RÉPONSES

OCTOBRE 1960 — NF 6

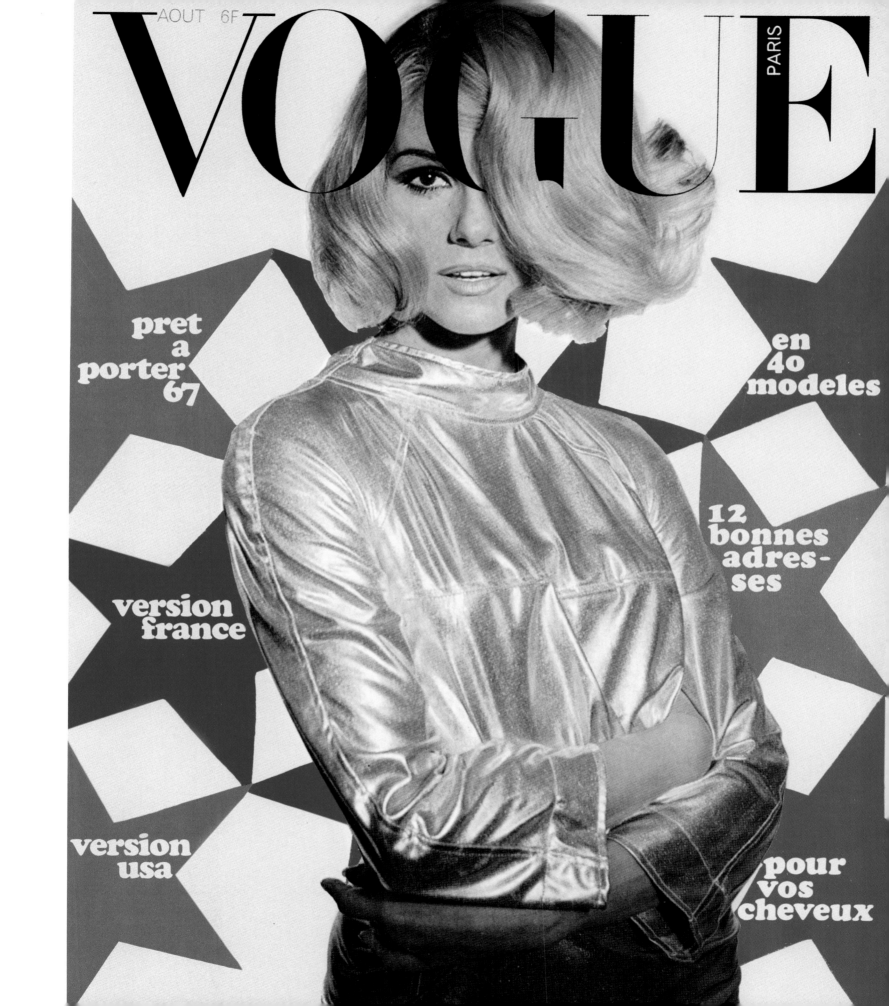

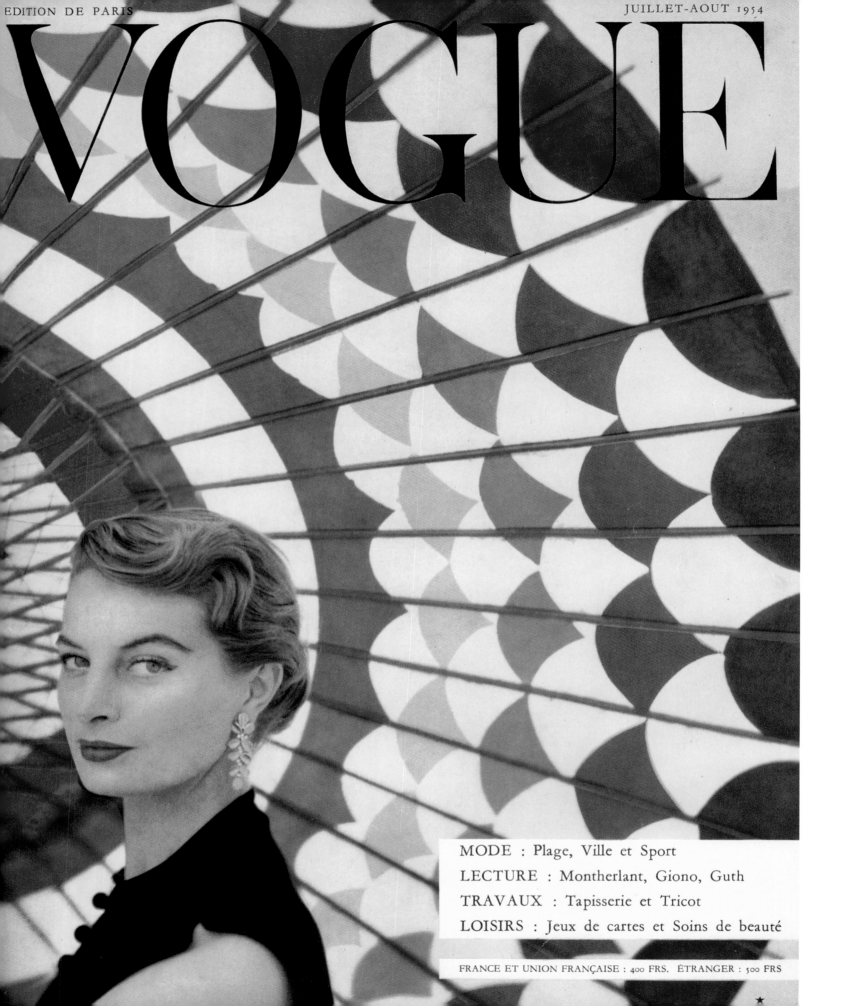

EDITION DE PARIS

JUILLET-AOUT 1954

VOGUE

MODE : Plage, Ville et Sport

LECTURE : Montherlant, Giono, Guth

TRAVAUX : Tapisserie et Tricot

LOISIRS : Jeux de cartes et Soins de beauté

FRANCE ET UNION FRANÇAISE : 400 FRS.   ÉTRANGER : 500 FRS

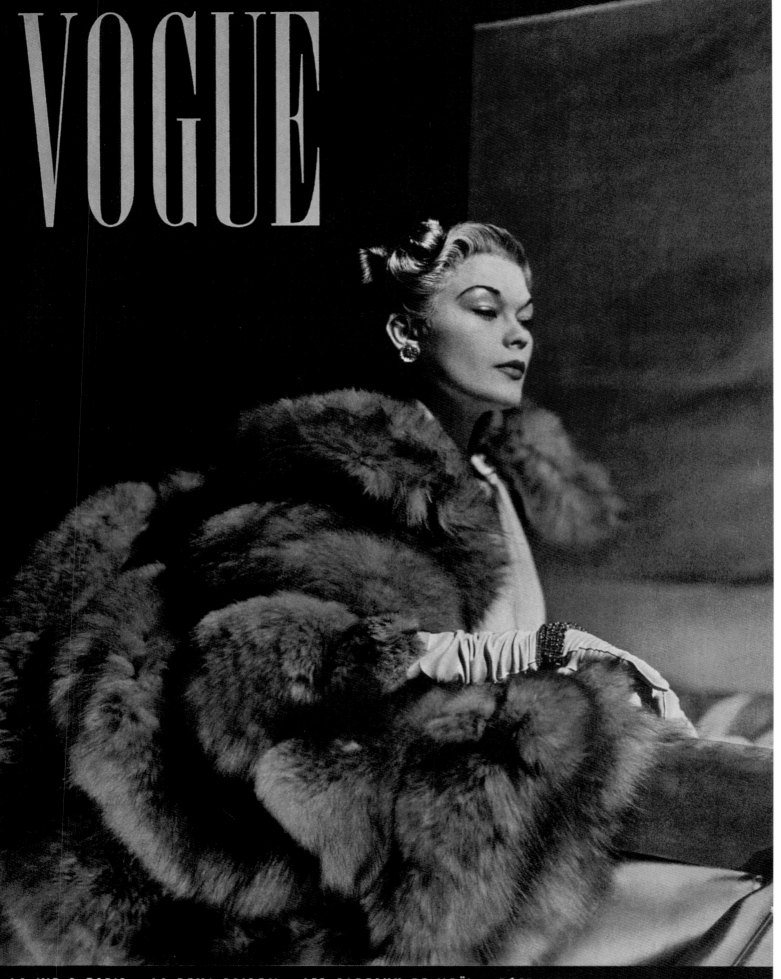

VOGUE

REVUE MENSUELLE LES ÉDITIONS CONDÉ NAST

LA VIE A PARIS • LA DEMI-SAISON • LES CADEAUX DE NOËL • DÉCEMBRE 1937 • PRIX 10 FRS

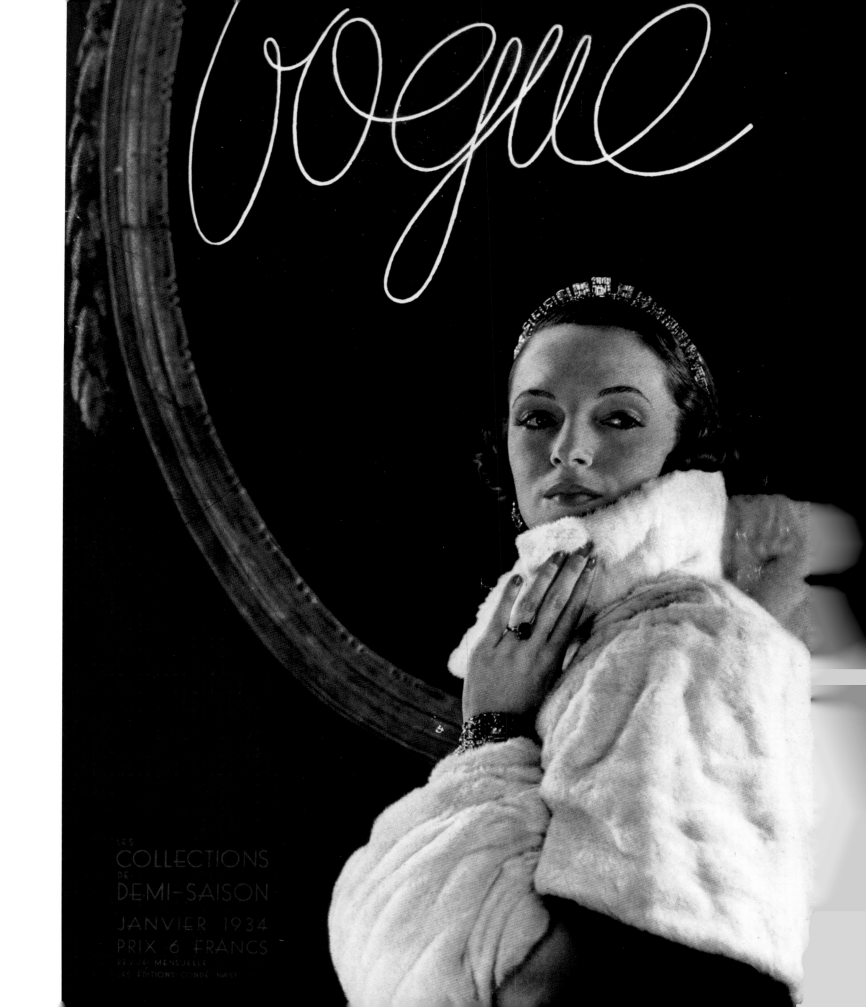

Vogue

LES
COLLECTIONS
DE
DEMI-SAISON

JANVIER 1934
PRIX 6 FRANCS
REVUE MENSUELLE
LES ÉDITIONS CONDÉ NAST

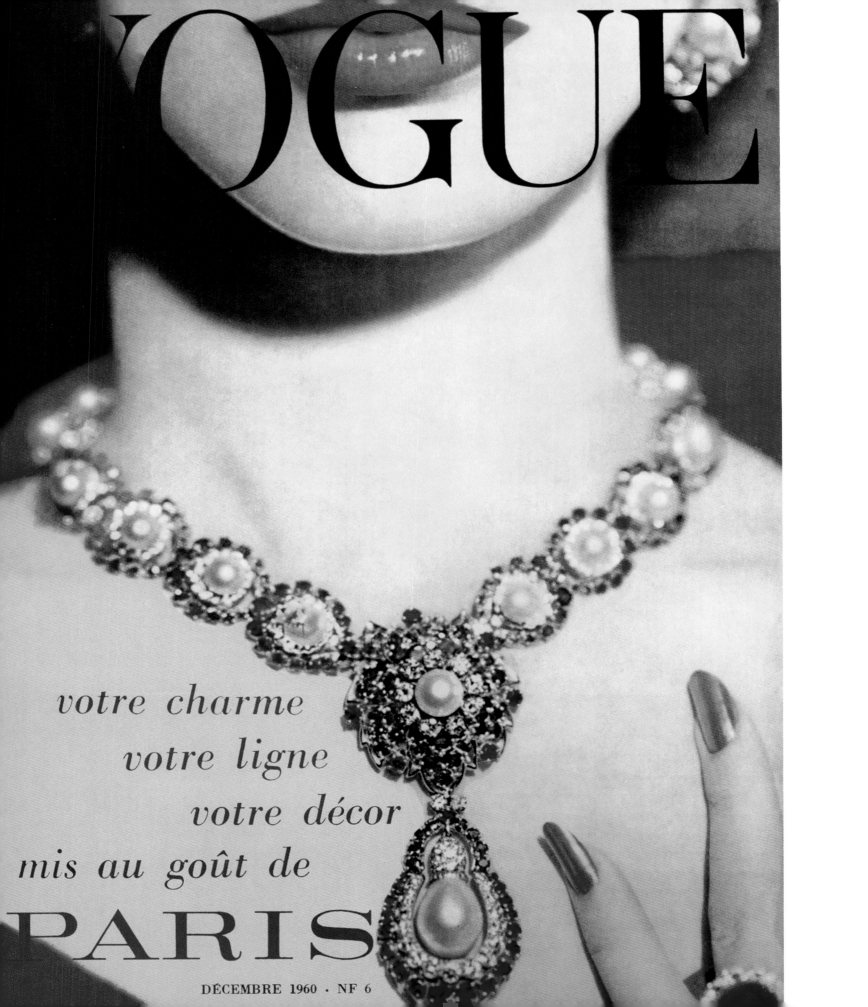

VOGUE

votre charme
votre ligne
votre décor
mis au goût de

PARIS

DÉCEMBRE 1960 · NF 6

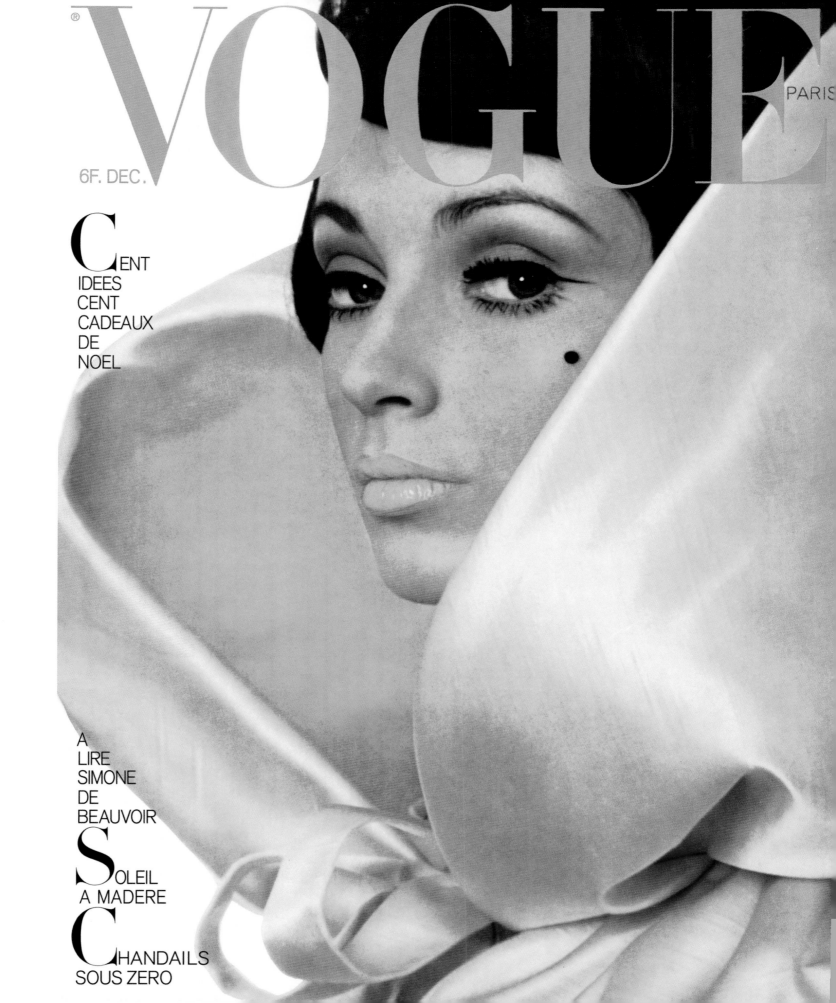

VOGUE

PARIS

®

6F. DEC.

Cent
IDEES
CENT
CADEAUX
DE
NOEL

A
LIRE
SIMONE
DE
BEAUVOIR

Soleil
A MADERE

Chandails
SOUS ZERO

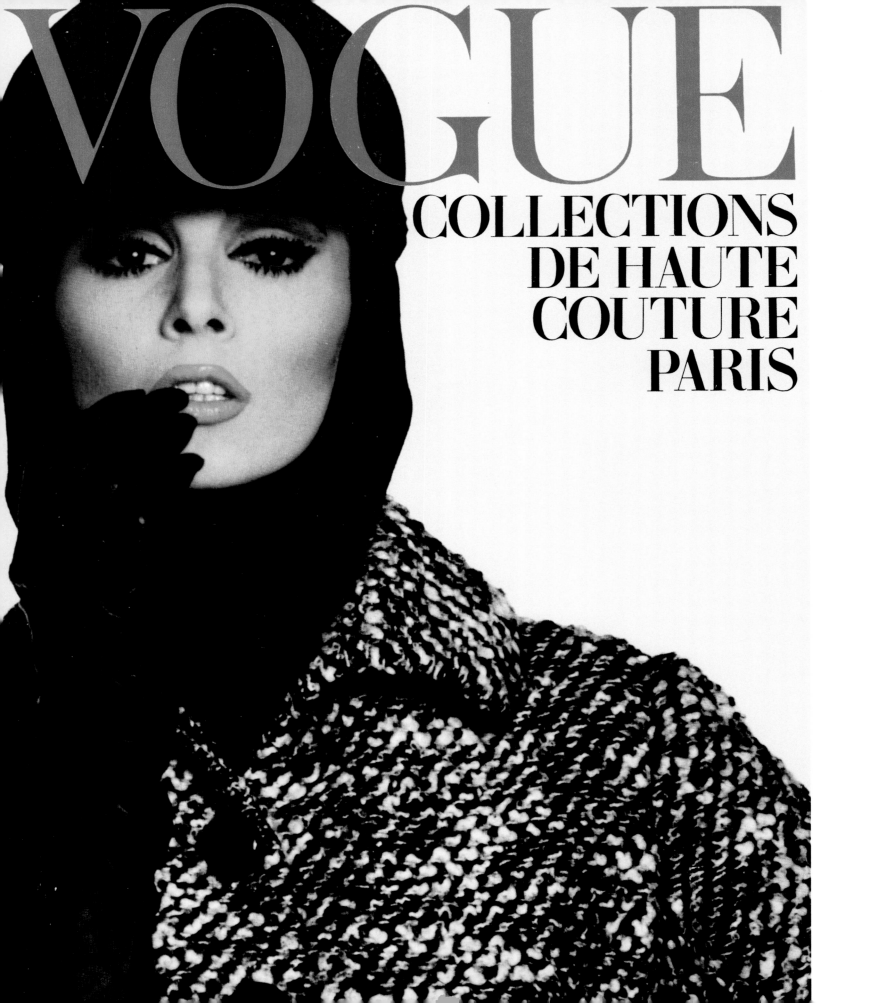

VOGUE

COLLECTIONS DE HAUTE COUTURE PARIS

Models and supermodels

'"Patience!" they said to me. "It's all going to change; the role
of the model is evolving... We couturiers will make her a loyal
collaborator; she'll be decently paid, precise, able to make a
steady living from her beauty and her grace..."'
— Colette, *Vogue*, April 1925

For most of the twentieth century, there was no such thing as a modelling agency, and
modelling itself could scarcely be described as a profession. The *maisons de couture*
had their own in-house models and muses, and magazines their own ways and means
of enlisting the services of the prettiest women and girls. At *Vogue*, this commissioning
flair was embodied in the person of Madame Dilé, known as 'Dilette' for short, whose
office was situated next to the studio. She was the person whose job it was to keep a
list of contacts and sometimes to identify new ones. Potential models were identified
at random, in the course of everyday business – beautiful or interesting women whom
the photographers and Dilette herself 'discovered' in restaurants and night clubs.
Persuading these women to model for *Vogue* was not always an easy matter, however:
not only were the fees offered modest, but many of the 'recruits' (who were often
from good backgrounds) feared the reaction of family and friends. Régine Destribaud,
who was to become one of Irving Penn's favourite models, was 'spotted' by *Vogue* in
1947 and recalls that she did not dare tell her parents about her collaboration with

the magazine for fear of shocking them. But, she continues, 'despite my family's reservations, I kept going and told my mother that it was to get a bit of pocket money and that, anyway, *Vogue* was the most elegant magazine around; the diplomatic corps of fashion…'[1]

Dilette was renowned for her unfailing instinct with regard to new recruits – a reputation that extended well beyond the walls of the *Vogue* office. She regularly received phone calls from other magazines asking for contacts, and it became the rule that new models had to agree to work exclusively for *Vogue* during the collections.

It was not until the 1980s, and more particularly the 1990s, that models began to acquire star status, becoming the heroines of the tabloids, the new goddesses of the celebrity stratosphere, fuelling our fantasies of beauty, fame and love. The most famous – Claudia, Naomi, Linda, Christy – earned serious money, attracting worldwide media attention. Did *Vogue* fuel this phenomenon? Not necessarily, or at any rate not consistently. When Brooke Shields, Jerry Hall, Eva Herzigova, Stephanie Seymour, Laetitia Casta and Claudia Schiffer grabbed the magazine's front page, the timing was often out: either they were not yet supermodels – Christy Turlington and Cindy Crawford were just starting out when Bill King photographed them in 1986 and 1987 respectively (during the great era of cover close-ups, taken preferably in the morning when the model was still fresh, and set off with satin and diamonds that were visible from afar) – or they had already acquired a degree of celebrity, experience and maturity and were chosen for their star status and presented accordingly. *Vogue* photographed them in the same manner that it photographed other stars, introducing an element of surprise or at any rate a different angle on the usual way they were presented. This was the case, for example, with Linda Evangelista in November 2001, Claudia Schiffer in April 2002, Laetitia Casta in September 2004, and Naomi Campbell and Kate Moss in April 2006.

Nevertheless, there does seem to be an ideal *Vogue* 'profile', which can be summed up as 'an attitude (Leslie Winer), unusual proportions (Kate Moss), a charming defect (the gap in Lauren Hutton's front teeth) or a strong character (Naomi). In each case, it amounts to an extra something which makes the image identifiable, and unforgettable', as we read in the February 2009 issue, on the front page of which the model Lara Stone shows off her 'devastating looks as opposed to classical beauty, her arousing figure, her Béatrice Dalle mouth and irreverent nature, all of which have charmed Paris *Vogue*'.

Vogue models are above all modern, whether they are already top models or not. Personality is what counts first and foremost. Never has it been purely a matter of flawlessly smooth looks, or a figure that is immaculately formed. But the power of the image is paramount. A name, however hallowed, is never enough to justify a cover, or to ensure the success of a particular issue: in October 2007, Gisele Bündchen, a star of international standing and an undisputed asset to the magazine, showed off her exceptional looks on the front cover, with a lagoon in the background. Commercially speaking, however, the sales figures fell below expectations. Was it because she was pictured too far away, and was not engaging the reader with her eyes? Did the image create an impression of aloofness? All we can say with certainty is that the weight given to personality, to a person who has the gift simultaneously to represent her age and to reflect her own individual difference, to embody, as it were, both the plural and the singular, is what characterizes the *Vogue* model. This is what governed the choice of Twiggy in May 1967 and of Lauren Hutton in October 1968, both of them strong characters, women who were neither completely different from everyone else nor completely the same.

In point of fact, Kate Moss remains the most exemplary of the magazine's contemporary icons, with far more covers to her name than most models and, in 2005, a Christmas edition entirely devoted to her. This is how Carine Roitfeld began her editorial for that issue: 'Kate Moss in a razor-cut platinum blonde bob, with her shoulder bare and her face in semi-profile, appeared on the cover of *Vogue* in February 2001. There's nothing very special about that, you may say, except that that *Vogue* was my first as Editor-in-Chief, and the choice of Kate to usher in a new era was not a matter of chance. With her height of barely one metre seventy (five feet seven inches), her adolescent looks and her absolute spontaneity, Kate, apart from being staggeringly photogenic, embodied a modernity and an accessibility we'd never seen before.'

In the wake of Kate Moss, number one *Vogue* model, have come a host of new faces, styles and characters to whom the magazine devoted a special issue in April 2008, among them Mariacarla Boscono, Natasha Poly, Sasha Pivovarova, Daria Werbowy, Lily Donaldson and Lara Stone – a new wave described by *Vogue* as 'no doubt quieter, certainly possessing less star status, but young, of mixed race, nomadic and on the move'. Watch this space…

1 Interview conducted by Susan Train in 1995.

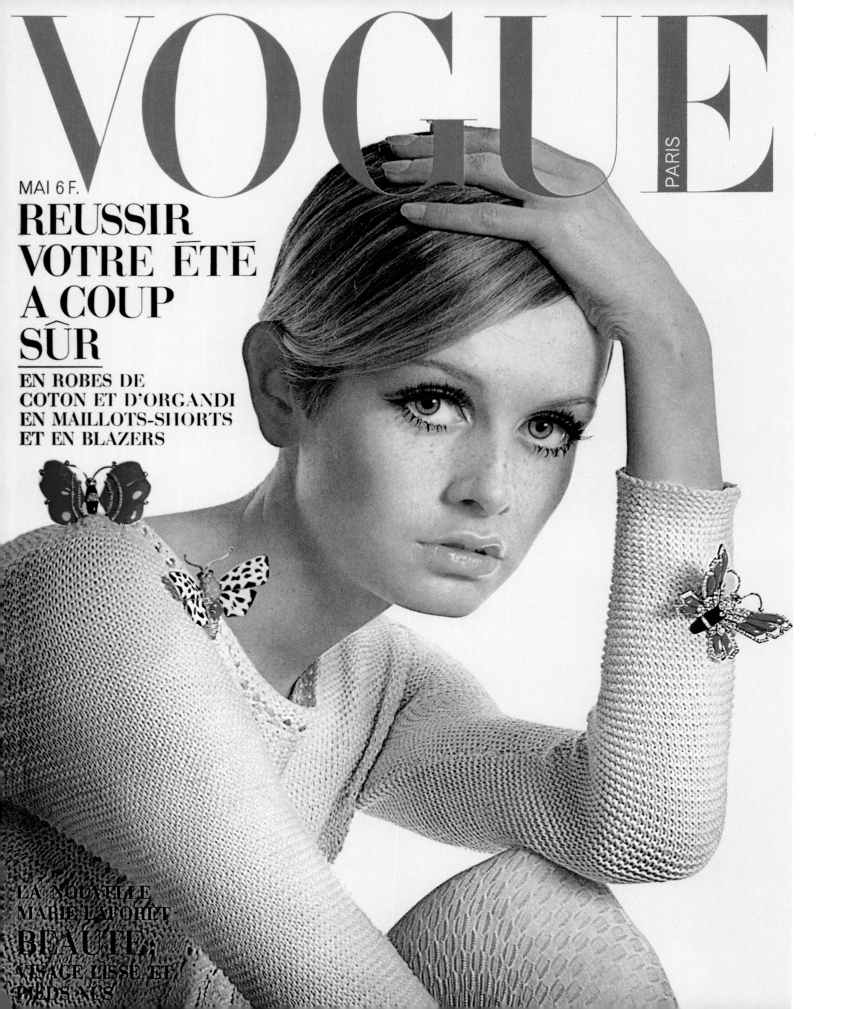

VOGUE

PARIS

MAI 6 F.

REUSSIR VOTRE ÉTÉ A COUP SÛR

EN ROBES DE
COTON ET D'ORGANDI
EN MAILLOTS-SHORTS
ET EN BLAZERS

LA NOUVELLE
MARIE LAFORÊT
BEAUTÉ
VISAGE LISSE ET
PIEDS NUS

May 1967
Henry Clarke
Model Twiggy

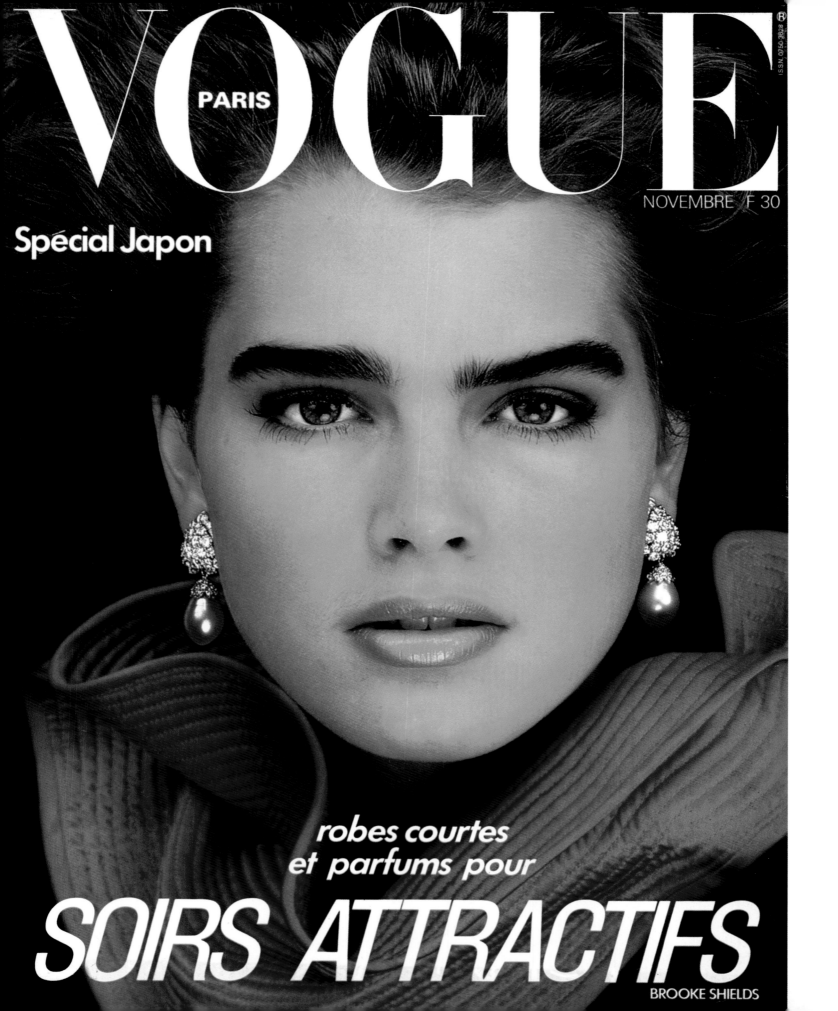

VOGUE

PARIS

NOVEMBRE F 30

Spécial Japon

ISSN 0750-3628

*robes courtes
et parfums pour*

SOIRS ATTRACTIFS

BROOKE SHIELDS

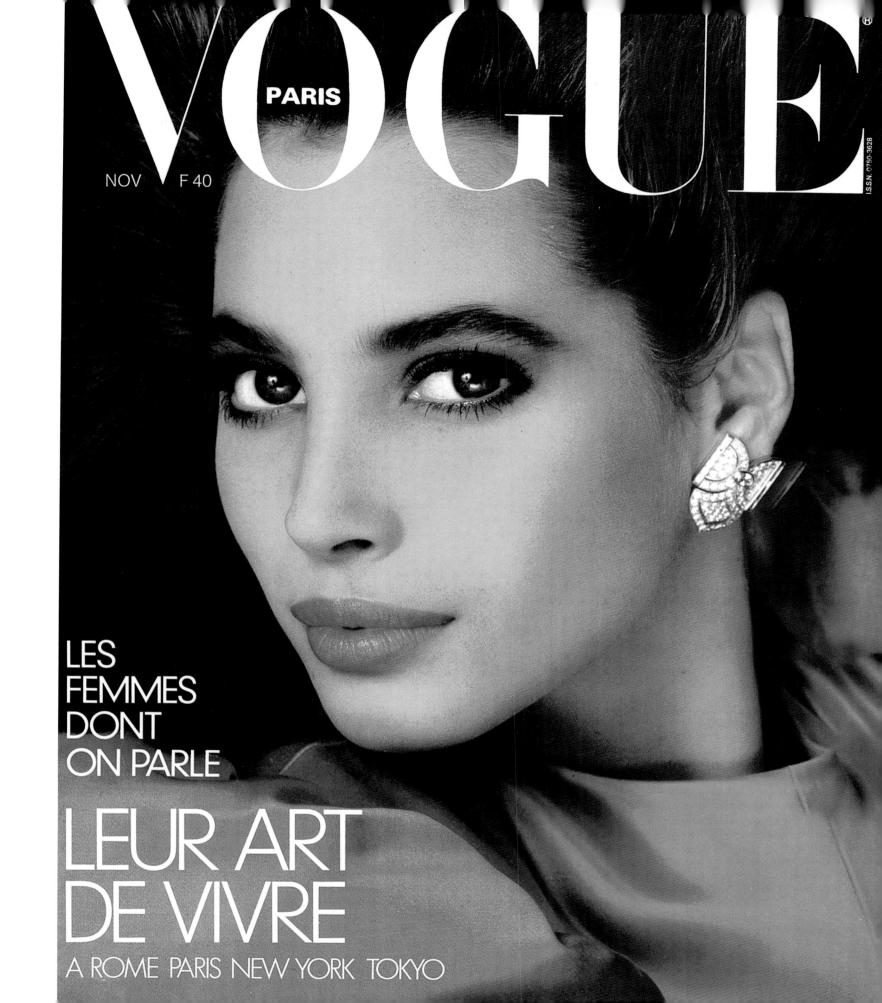

VOGUE

PARIS

NOV F 40

LES
FEMMES
DONT
ON PARLE

LEUR ART
DE VIVRE

A ROME PARIS NEW YORK TOKYO

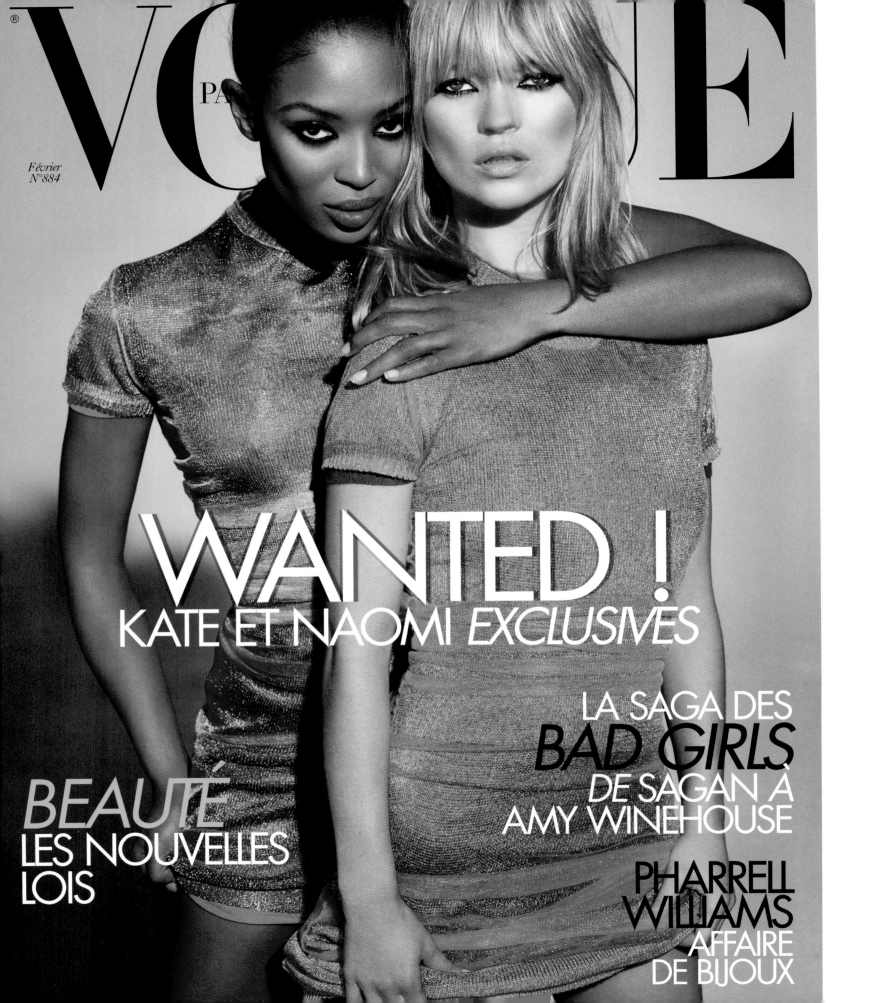

VOGUE

PARIS

Février
N°884

WANTED !
KATE ET NAOMI *EXCLUSIVES*

LA SAGA DES
BAD GIRLS
DE SAGAN À
AMY WINEHOUSE

BEAUTÉ
LES NOUVELLES
LOIS

PHARRELL
WILLIAMS
AFFAIRE
DE BIJOUX

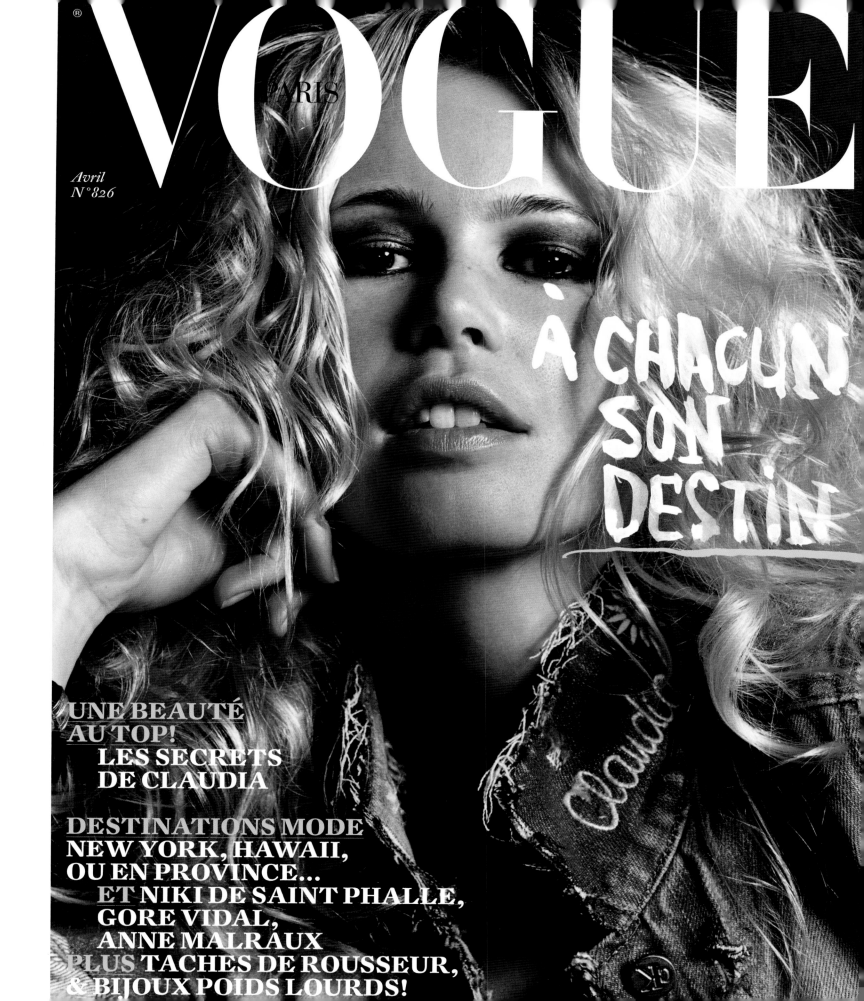

VOGUE

PARIS

Avril
N°826

À CHACUN SON DESTIN

**UNE BEAUTÉ
AU TOP!**
LES SECRETS
DE CLAUDIA

DESTINATIONS MODE
NEW YORK, HAWAII,
OU EN PROVINCE...
ET NIKI DE SAINT PHALLE,
GORE VIDAL,
ANNE MALRAUX
PLUS TACHES DE ROUSSEUR,
& BIJOUX POIDS LOURDS!

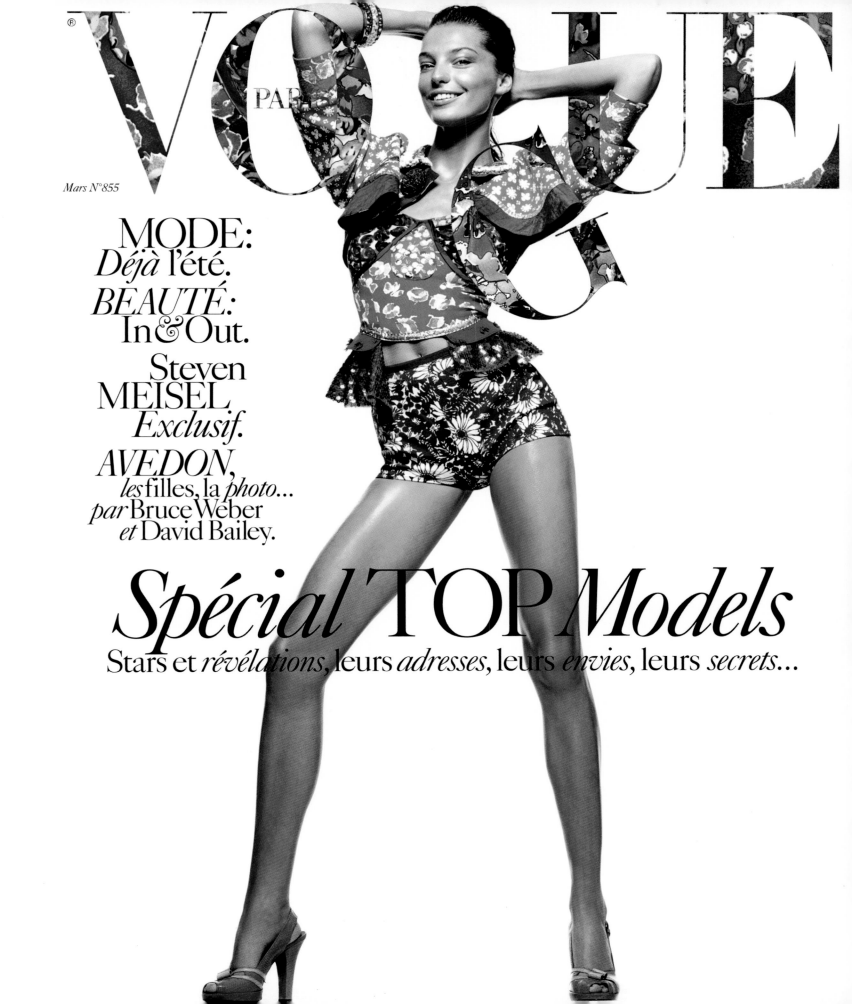

VOGUE

PARIS

Mars N°855

MODE:
Déjà l'été.
BEAUTÉ:
In & Out.
Steven
MEISEL
Exclusif.
AVEDON,
les filles, la *photo…*
par Bruce Weber
et David Bailey.

Spécial TOP *Models*
Stars et *révélations,* leurs *adresses,* leurs *envies,* leurs *secrets…*

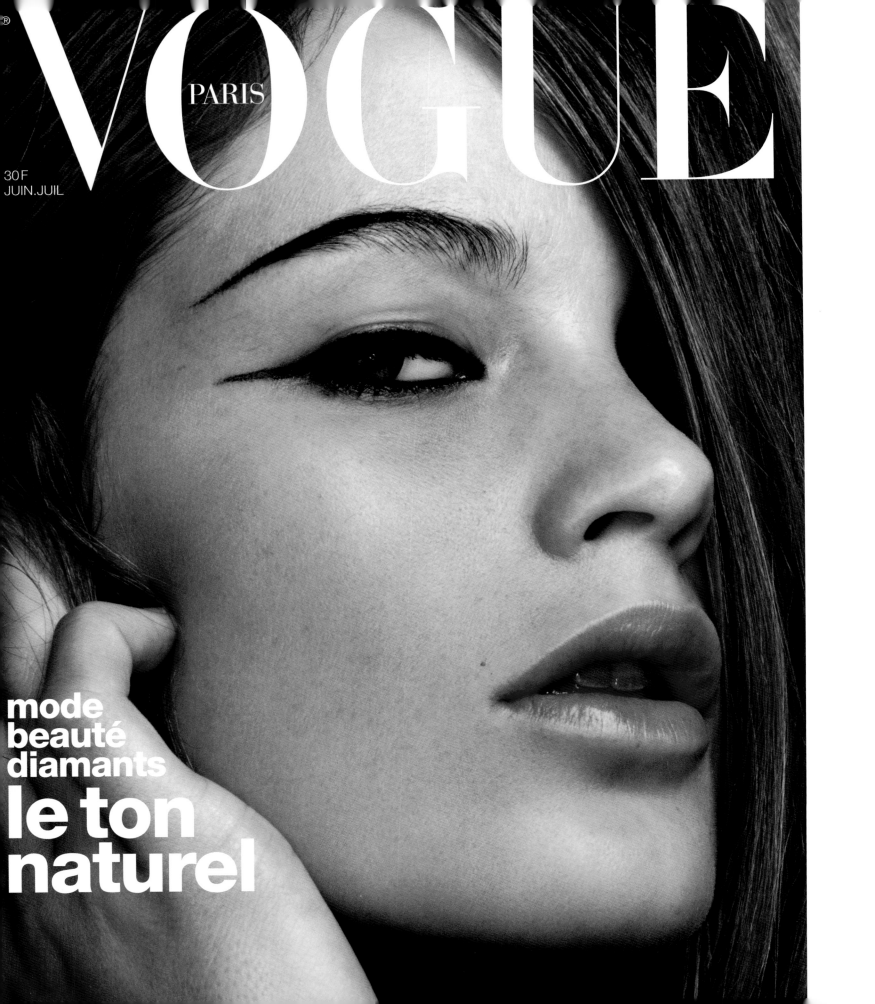

VOGUE

PARIS

30 F
JUIN.JUIL

mode
beauté
diamants
**le ton
naturel**

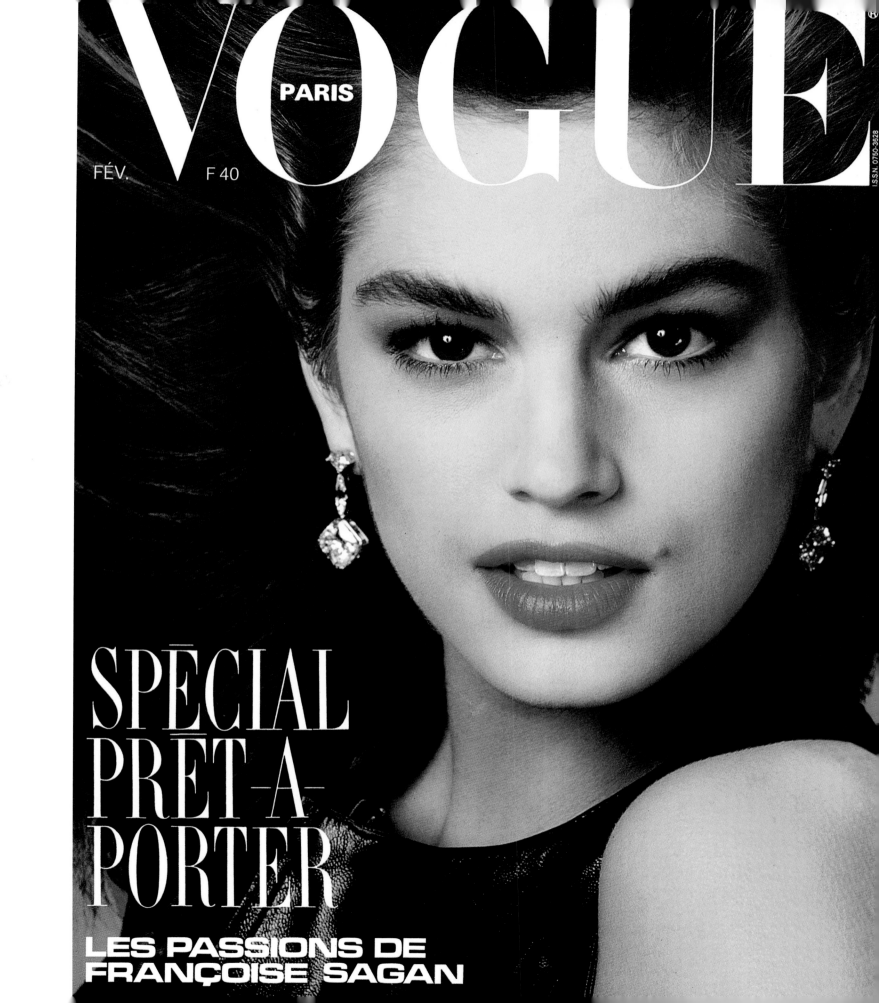

VOGUE

PARIS

FÉV. F 40

J.S.S.N. 0750-3628

SPÉCIAL
PRÊT-A-
PORTER

LES PASSIONS DE
FRANÇOISE SAGAN

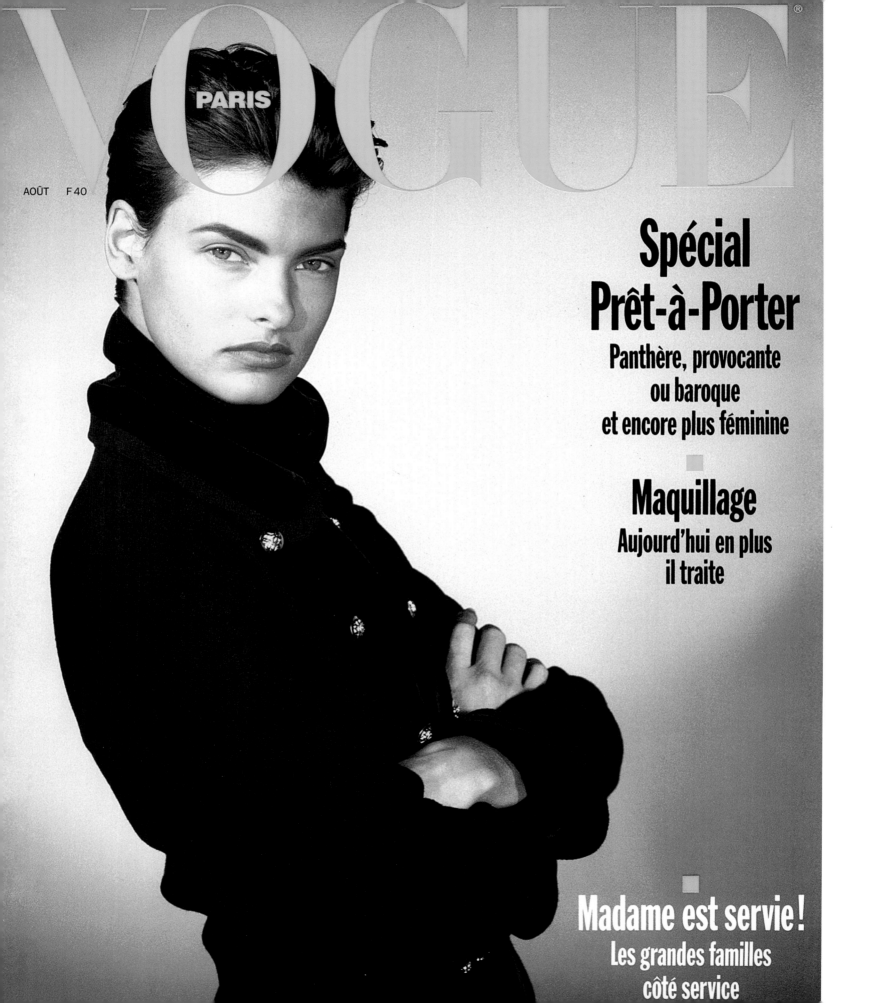

VOGUE

PARIS

AOÛT   F 40

Spécial
Prêt-à-Porter
Panthère, provocante
ou baroque
et encore plus féminine

Maquillage
Aujourd'hui en plus
il traite

Madame est servie !
Les grandes familles
côté service

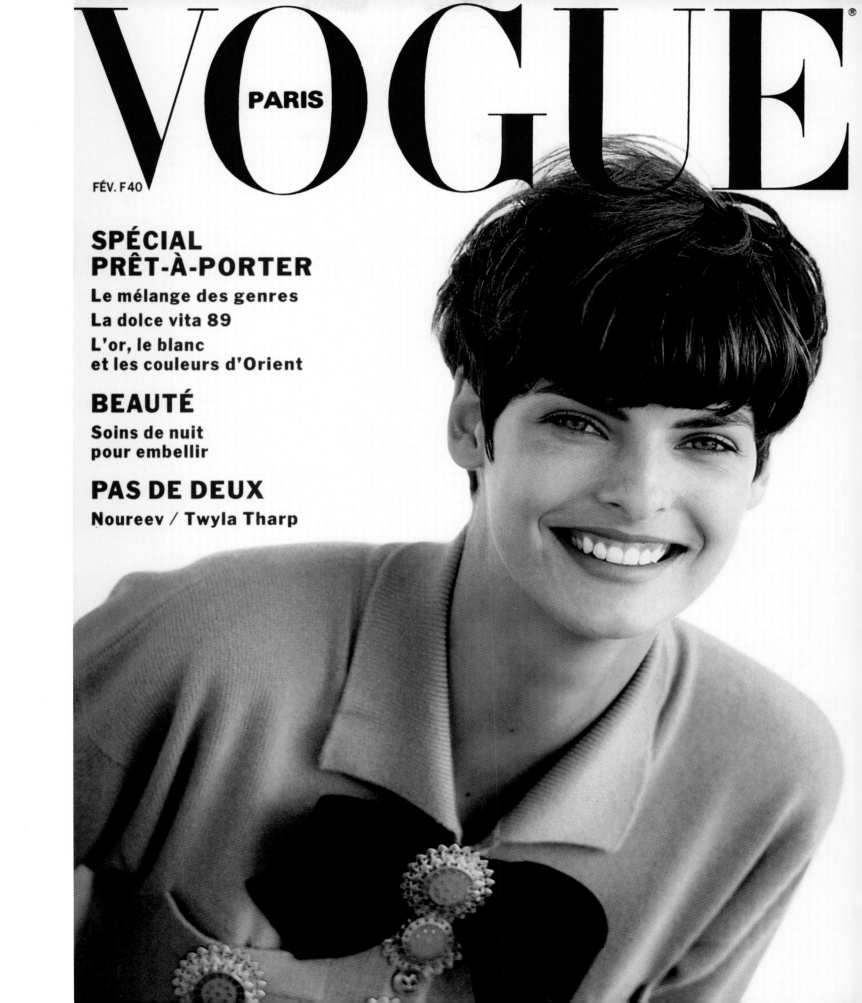

VOGUE PARIS

FÉV. F 40

SPÉCIAL PRÊT-À-PORTER

Le mélange des genres

La dolce vita 89

L'or, le blanc
et les couleurs d'Orient

BEAUTÉ

Soins de nuit
pour embellir

PAS DE DEUX

Noureev / Twyla Tharp

PREVIOUS PAGES
June–July 2001
Mario Testino
Model Carolyn Murphy

February 1987
Bill King
Model Cindy Crawford

August 1989
Steven Meisel
Model Linda Evangelista
Couturier Chanel

February 1989
Peter Lindbergh
Model Linda Evangelista

OPPOSITE
March 2004
David Sims
Model Kate Moss
Couturier Gucci

VOGUE

PARIS

Mars N° 845

STAR attitude
Spécial mode & beauté : or, paillettes, strass, soir...
...us les secrets pour briller.

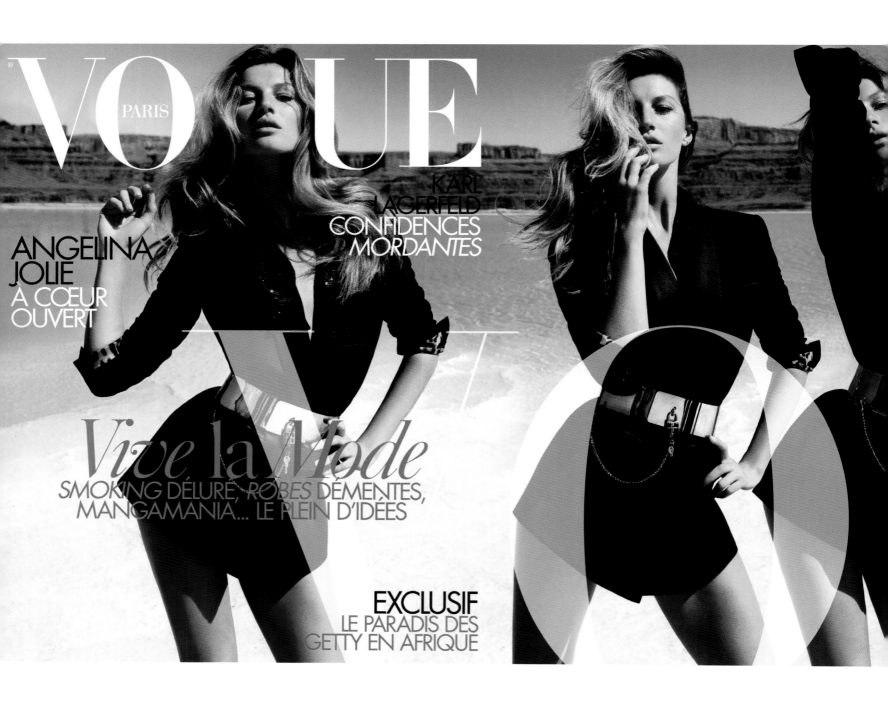

VOGUE

PARIS

ANGELINA
JOLIE
A CŒUR
OUVERT

KARL
LAGERFELD
CONFIDENCES
MORDANTES

Vive la Mode
SMOKING DÉLURÉ, ROBES DÉMENTES,
MANGAMANIA... LE PLEIN D'IDÉES

EXCLUSIF
LE PARADIS DES
GETTY EN AFRIQUE

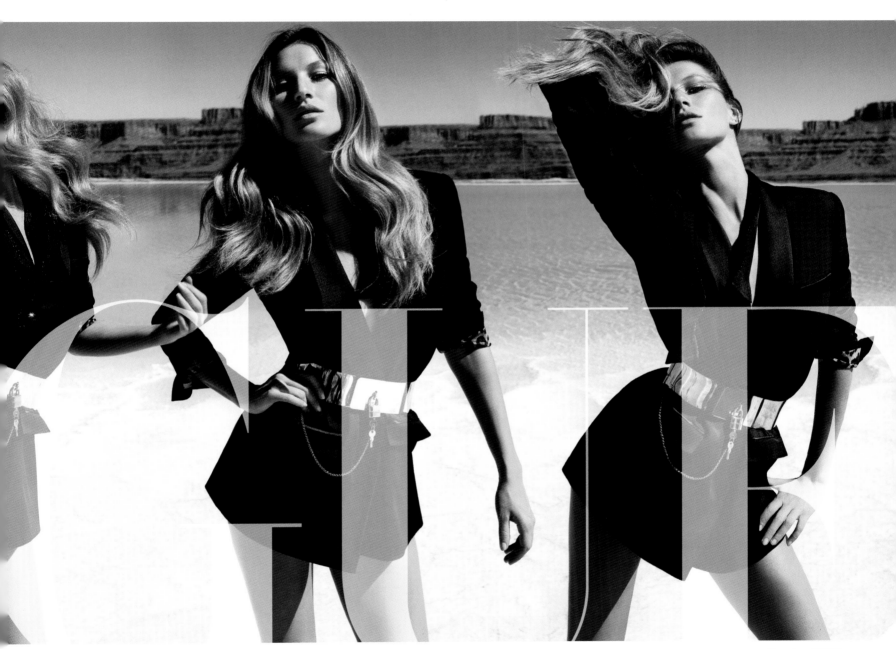

October 2007
Inez van Lamsweerde
& Vinoodh Matadin
Model Gisele Bündchen
Couturier Dolce & Gabbana

VOGUE

PARIS

F 40 SEPTEMBRE

JERRY HALL

HAUTE
COUTURE
CLIP SUR LES
COLLECTIONS

I.S.S.N 0750.3628

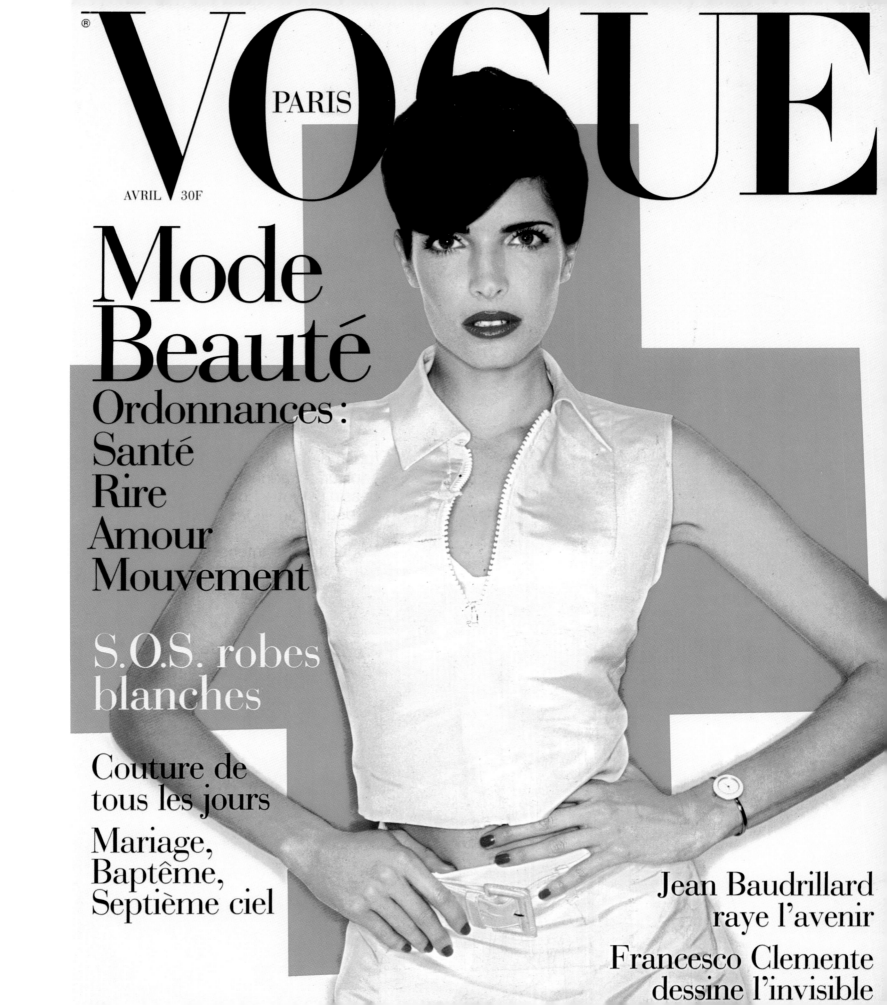

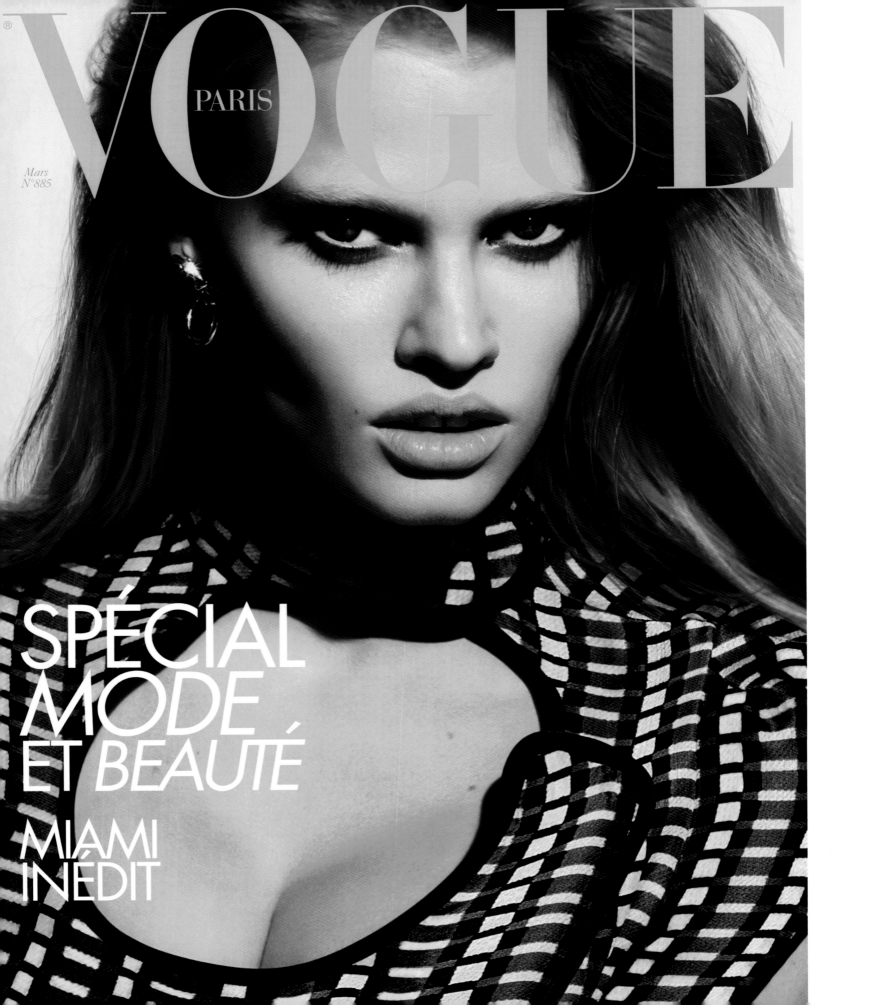

VOGUE
PARIS

Mars
N°885

SPÉCIAL
MODE
ET *BEAUTÉ*

MIAMI
INÉDIT

Hats off!

'A woman was asking me to explain and I said to her:
Explain your hat to me.'
— Jean Cocteau, *Journal* (1942–45)

The story goes that a member of American *Vogue*'s editorial staff tried to commit suicide by throwing herself under a subway train. After the dust had settled, Edna Woolman Chase supposedly gave her a little lecture, saying: 'We at *Vogue* don't throw ourselves under subway trains, my dear. If we must, we take sleeping pills.' Whether or not the anecdote is true, it speaks volumes.

Edna Woolman Chase was Editor-in-Chief of American *Vogue* from 1914 to 1952, and all the more influential because in those days a great many pages were common to all three editions of the magazine. But Paris remained the nerve centre of haute couture, the location where most of *Vogue*'s fashion stories were conceived, and either Edna herself or a member of her team were always there for the collections. She stipulated a strict dress code, requiring that her colleagues all wear a hat, white gloves and black stockings in public. And it would have been unthinkable to photograph a model with a cigarette in her hand. Behind the scenes at *Vogue*, people were expected to behave with the same impeccable manners and attention to their appearance as the magazine's elite readership – though that came naturally to the likes of the Princesse Bibesco who wrote the editorials for French *Vogue* and the Duchesse d'Ayen who held the fashion reins. These examples serve to remind us to what extent the people who advised on style, from the editorial heart of the magazine, were also the first to follow their own recommendations. There is nothing surprising, therefore, in the fact that, both in its pages and on its covers, *Vogue* accorded particular importance to hats, which, up until the 1950s, were not just a chic accessory but an indicator of savoir-faire. (It is worth remembering that Coco Chanel and Jeanne Lanvin were both milliners before becoming top couturiers.)

Hats had played a special role during the Occupation in Paris, when wearing one became a symbol of defiance against the Germans, an extravagant challenge to the rigours of the law and the privations of everyday life. Made of scraps of fabric and any other assorted materials that could be found, these hats were the expression of an unstoppable creative energy, a small bid for freedom. It was out of the question that *Vogue* could go on publishing under the watchful eye of the Germans, even less that it might collaborate, so the magazine closed its doors during this period; but when it started up again, hats were immediately on the agenda. In the Winter 1945–46 issue, we read: 'We have seen her [the Parisienne] these latter years, proudly sporting plumed jardinières, montgolfiers crowned with taffeta, structures bedecked with ribbons in acid hues and all the excesses involved in such an attention to style.'

After the Liberation, however, the hat and the great names associated with it – Paulette, Claude Saint-Cyr, Orcel, Reboux and Legroux Sœurs, for example – became the subject of at times heated debate among *Vogue*'s editors. At the start of the 1950s, hats came to be seen as festive accoutrements rather than ingredients of everyday wear. As time went by, they gradually came to be reserved for the races, for weddings and other special occasions, a development paralleled by the growing focus on hair, as women took increasing pleasure in experimenting with different cuts and styles. Hats were also worn less often by members of the *Vogue* team themselves, and Edmonde Charles-Roux, who joined the magazine in 1947 and became Editor-in-Chief in 1954, recalls that she was criticized for never wearing one: 'Michel de Brunhoff was very keen on supporting milliners and the millinery business, defending them at all costs and arguing that we could not allow an industry to die out; so we continued to promote them in the magazine, even though there were fewer and fewer in the high street. No one would have even dreamed of photographing an haute couture model without her matching hat, although the milliners actually criticized us for this, since they thought we were letting them down by favouring the couture labels…'[1]

This whole question of the hat reflects the close relationship that existed at the time between *Vogue* and the world of fashion. Edmonde Charles-Roux explains: 'Michel de Brunhoff was incredibly knowledgeable about haute couture. He was intimately acquainted with the work and the skills involved and he was a close friend of a number of couturiers, including Madeleine Vionnet, Elsa Schiaparelli, Robert Piguet, Lucien Lelong and Christian Dior. Dior called Michel several times a day and showed him his designs. We knew his models before the collection had even been put together – which demonstrates a marvellous level of trust. It was Michel, too, who took the young Yves Saint Laurent over to Dior's. He was in a position to do it and he could be absolutely sure that it was the right thing to do. *Vogue* was hugely influential in those days, and even more so in the 1930s. Abroad, it was read by all the ambassadors' wives. It set the tone for them. They would identify the designs they liked and call up the couture houses to speak to the sales assistants, whose role was crucial. They would telephone from the four corners of the globe, knowing exactly what they wanted, thanks to the fashion pages. These three – couturier, sales assistant and *Vogue* – formed a fantastically powerful trio in commercial terms: no one has any idea today.'

Michel de Brunhoff was a pivotal figure and a pillar of French haute couture, which he clandestinely promoted during the war. He had close links with the couture houses and was always eager to defend their industries. In the first post-war issue of *Vogue*, entitled 'Libération' and dated January 1945, the fashion pages opened with what sounds very like a manifesto: 'Let us never forget that Parisian haute couture provides a source of income for several hundreds of thousands of French people and that it occupies a central place in the export industries upon which the economic recovery of our country depends.' Brunhoff remained anxious to continue devoting space to hats, even at a time when they were falling out of fashion. He had his allies, too, in particular Guy Bourdin, who was especially fond of featuring hats in his photographs.

The hats we see splashed across the covers of *Vogue* thus tell a number of stories down the years: the indispensable class badge of the 1920s and 1930s, hats became the symbol of creative defiance in 1940s occupied France, manifestos of couture skill in the 1950s, instances of dressy or eccentric style and something of a rarity in the 1960s, the expression of a photographer's whim no less than of fashion. From the 1980s onwards, they appeared only very sporadically, sometimes as symbols of defiance, but always contributing to a sensational image, an attention-grabbing element but also a respectful nod in the direction of artistic creativity, reminding us that *Vogue* has always sought to promote individuality no less than excellence.

1 Interview conducted by Susan Train in 1995.

August 1936
Horst P. Horst
Hat by Molyneux

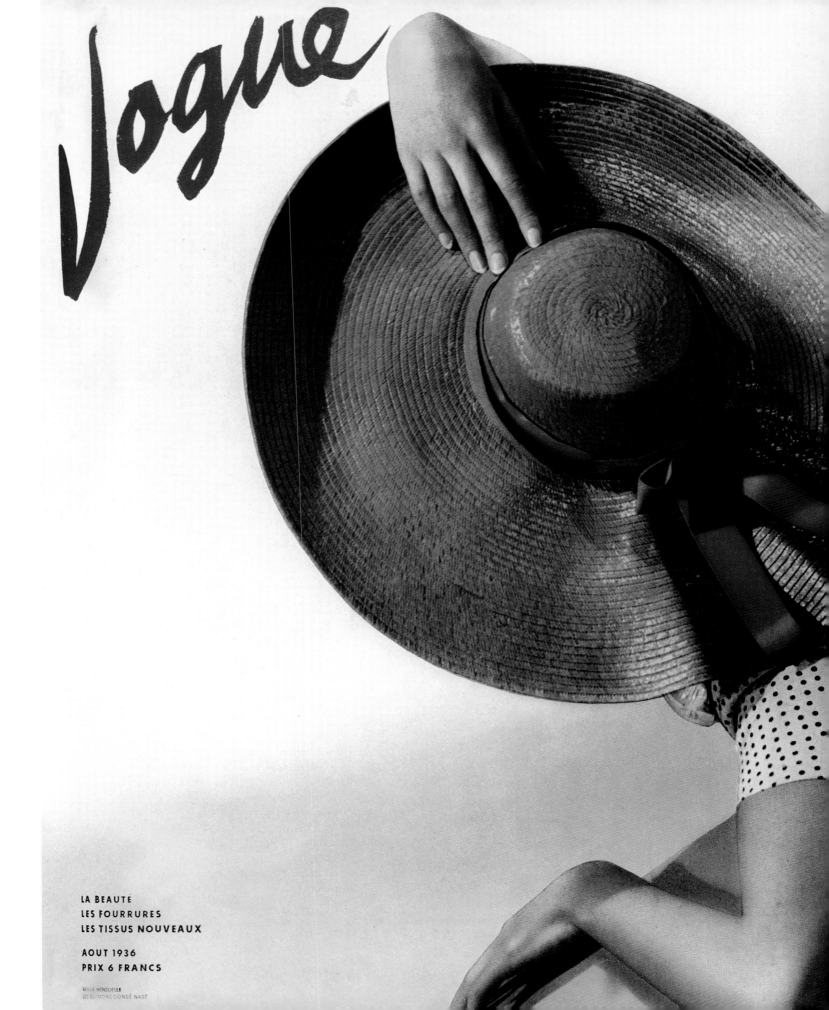

Vogue

LA BEAUTÉ
LES FOURRURES
LES TISSUS NOUVEAUX

AOUT 1936
PRIX 6 FRANCS

REVUE MENSUELLE
LES ÉDITIONS CONDÉ NAST

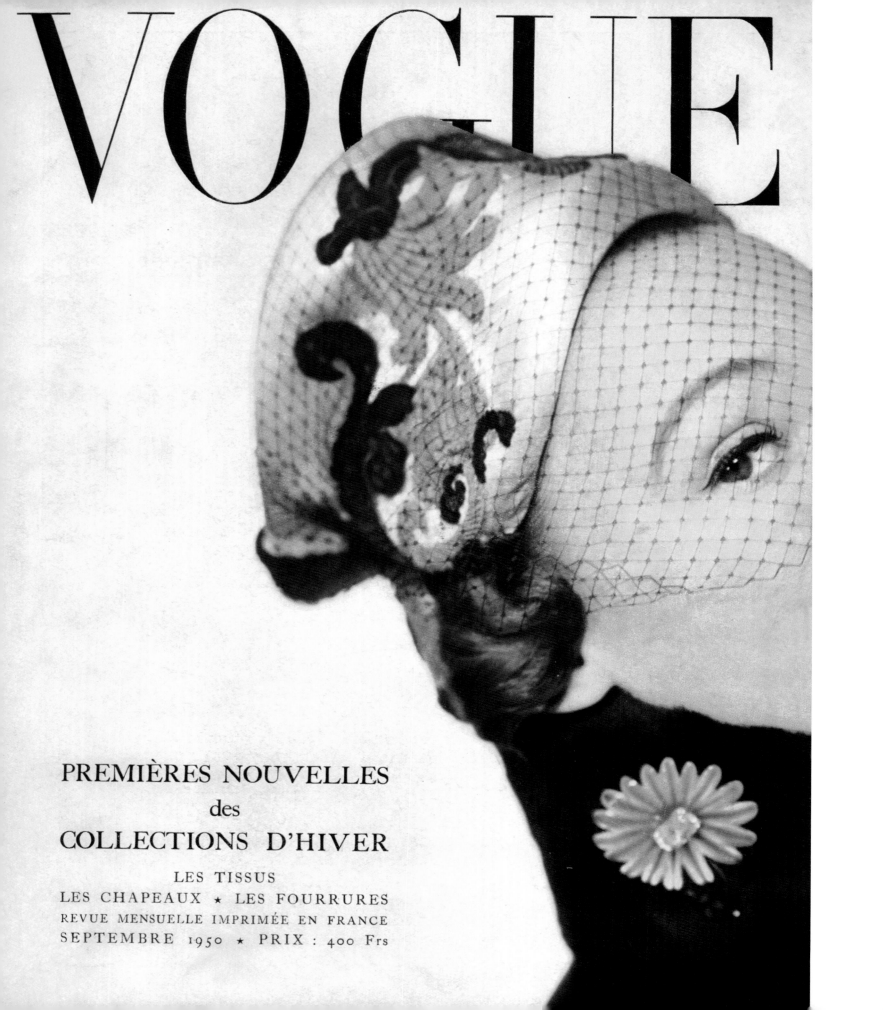

VOGUE

PREMIÈRES NOUVELLES

des

COLLECTIONS D'HIVER

LES TISSUS

LES CHAPEAUX ★ LES FOURRURES

REVUE MENSUELLE IMPRIMÉE EN FRANCE

SEPTEMBRE 1950 ★ PRIX : 400 Frs

VOGUE

UNE GRANDE ENQUÊTE : BEAUTÉ D'ÉTÉ
MAQUILLAGE DOUX
PRODUITS NATURELS
NOUVELLES CRÈMES DE SOINS

POUR ÊTRE MINCE :
LE RÉGIME DES VACANCES

POUR ÊTRE A LA PAGE :
TOUS LES MAILLOTS

ET LE SUPPLÉMENT VOGUE-EUROPE   JUIN-JUILLET 1961 · NF 6

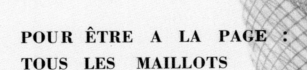

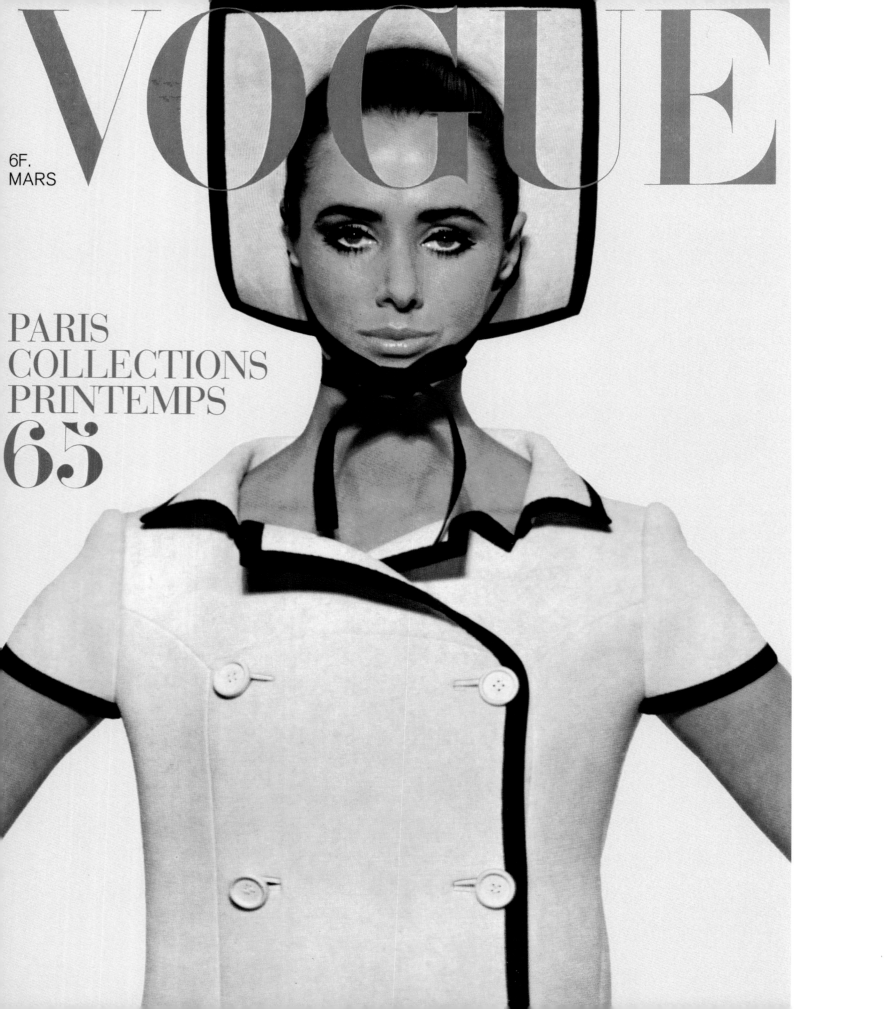

VOGUE

6F.
MARS

PARIS
COLLECTIONS
PRINTEMPS
65

VOGUE

AVRIL 1951   REVUE MENSUELLE • IMPRIMÉE EN FRANCE   500 FRANCS

NUMÉRO SPÉCIAL

DES

COLLECTIONS DE PRINTEMPS

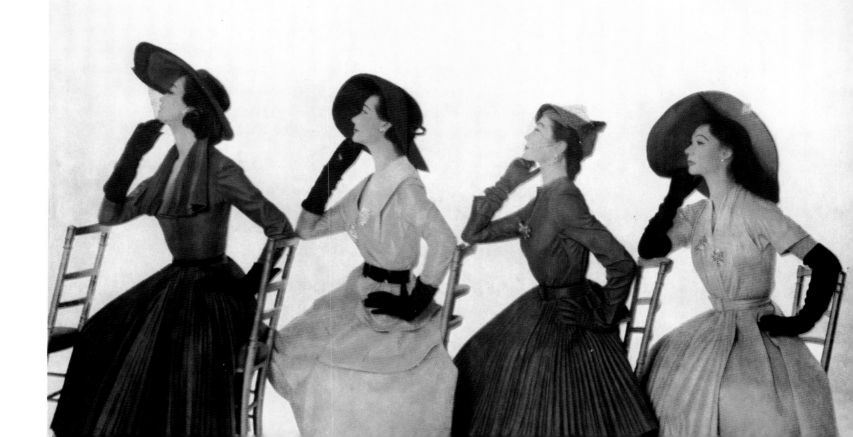

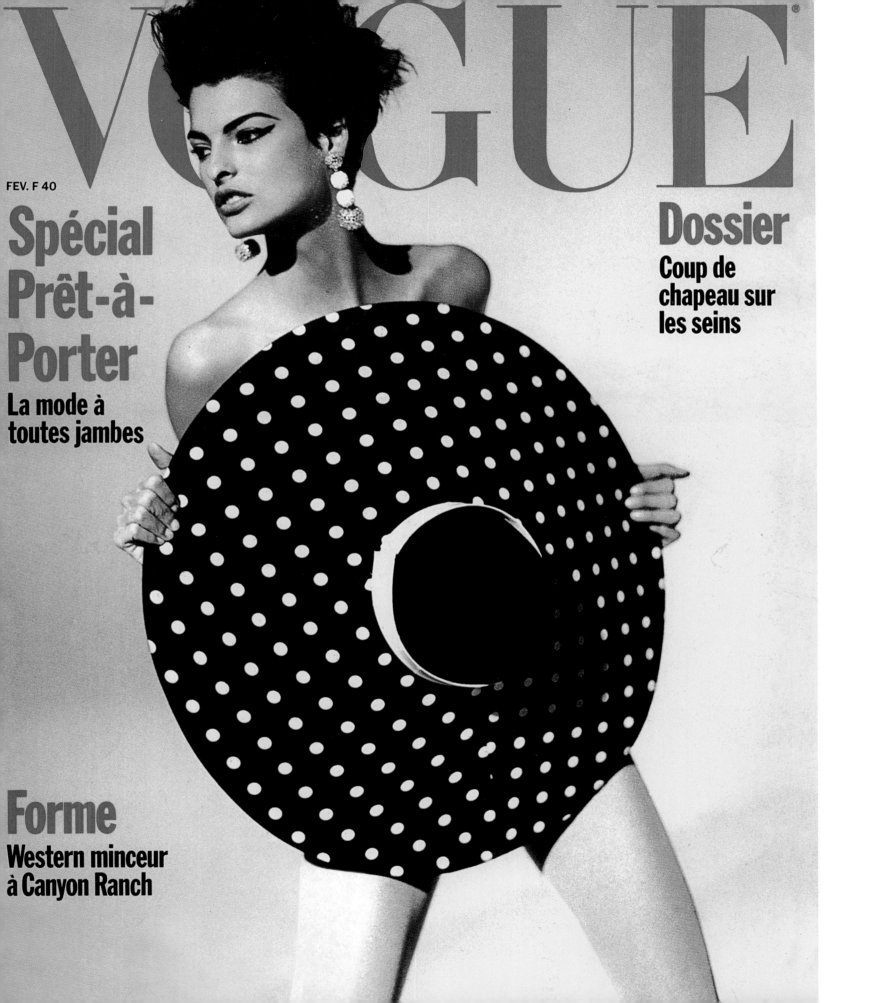

VOGUE

FEV. F 40

Spécial Prêt-à-Porter

La mode à toutes jambes

Dossier

Coup de chapeau sur les seins

Forme

Western minceur à Canyon Ranch

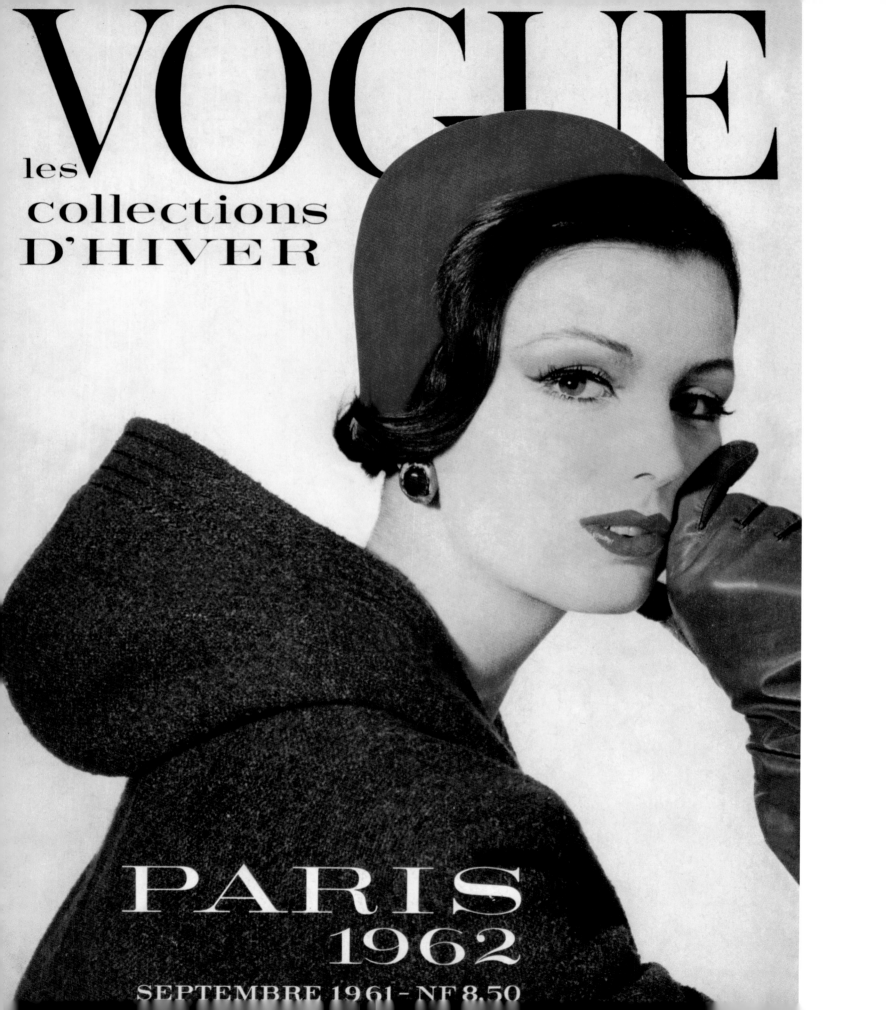

VOGUE

les collections D'HIVER

PARIS
1962

SEPTEMBRE 1961 - NF 8,50

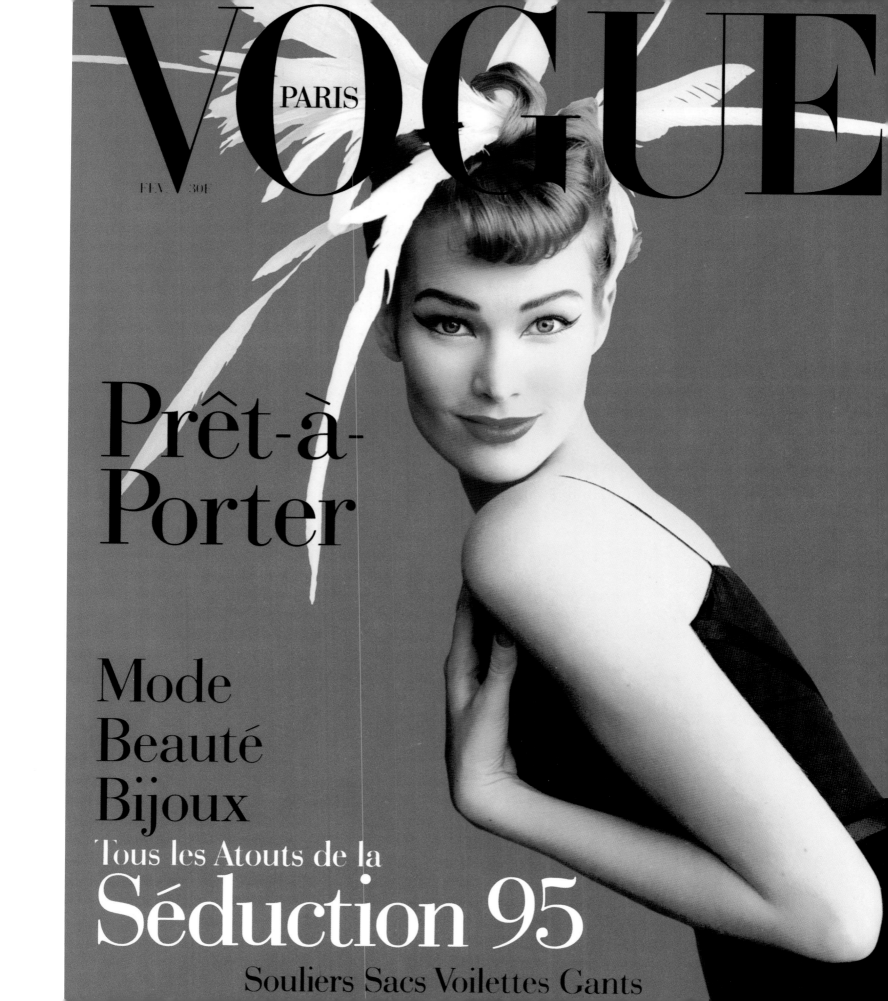

VOGUE
PARIS

FÉV 30F

Prêt-à-Porter

Mode
Beauté
Bijoux

Tous les Atouts de la
Séduction 95

Souliers Sacs Voilettes Gants

VOGUE

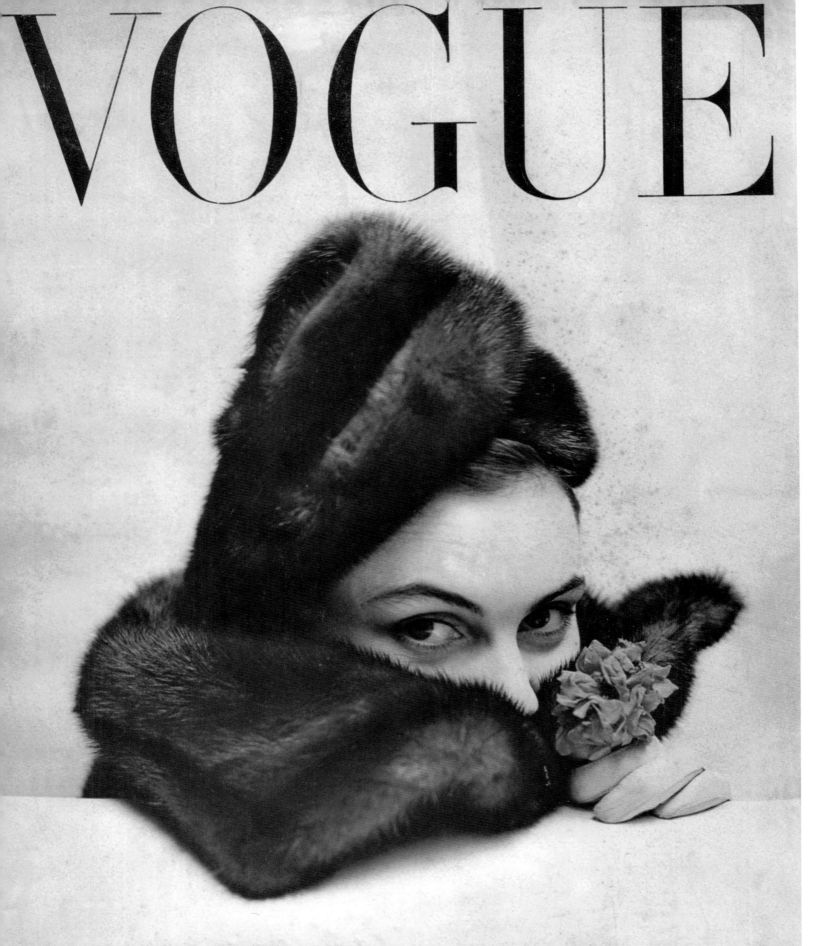

LA MODE D'HIVER · LES FOURRURES

Novembre 1949 - Revue Mensuelle - Imprimée en France - Prix: 350 frs

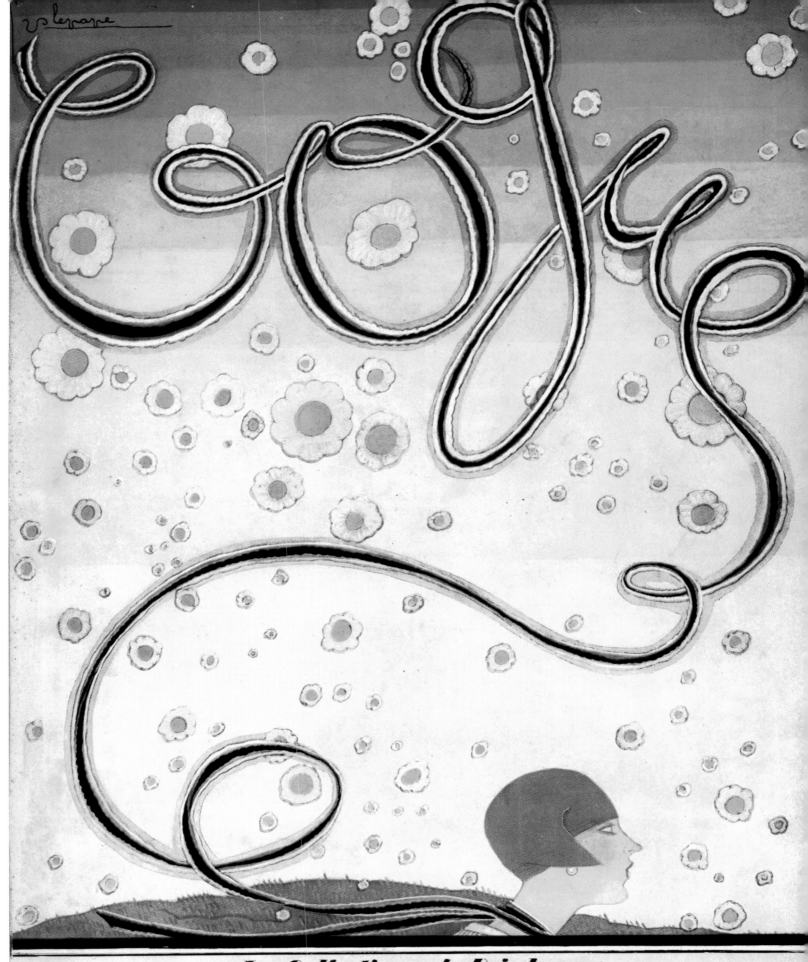

Vogue

Les Collections de Printemps

Revue Mensuelle

LES ÉDITIONS CONDÉ NAST

AVRIL 1928

PRIX: 6 FRCS.

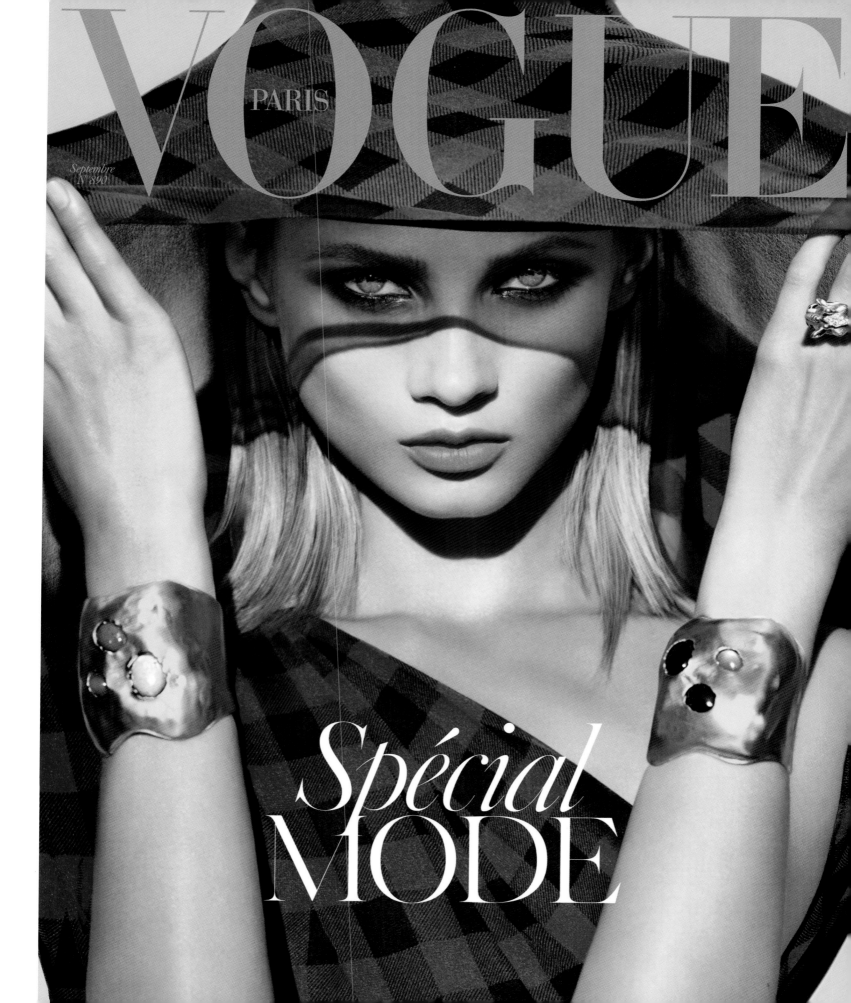

VOGUE

PARIS

Septembre
Nº 890

Spécial
MODE

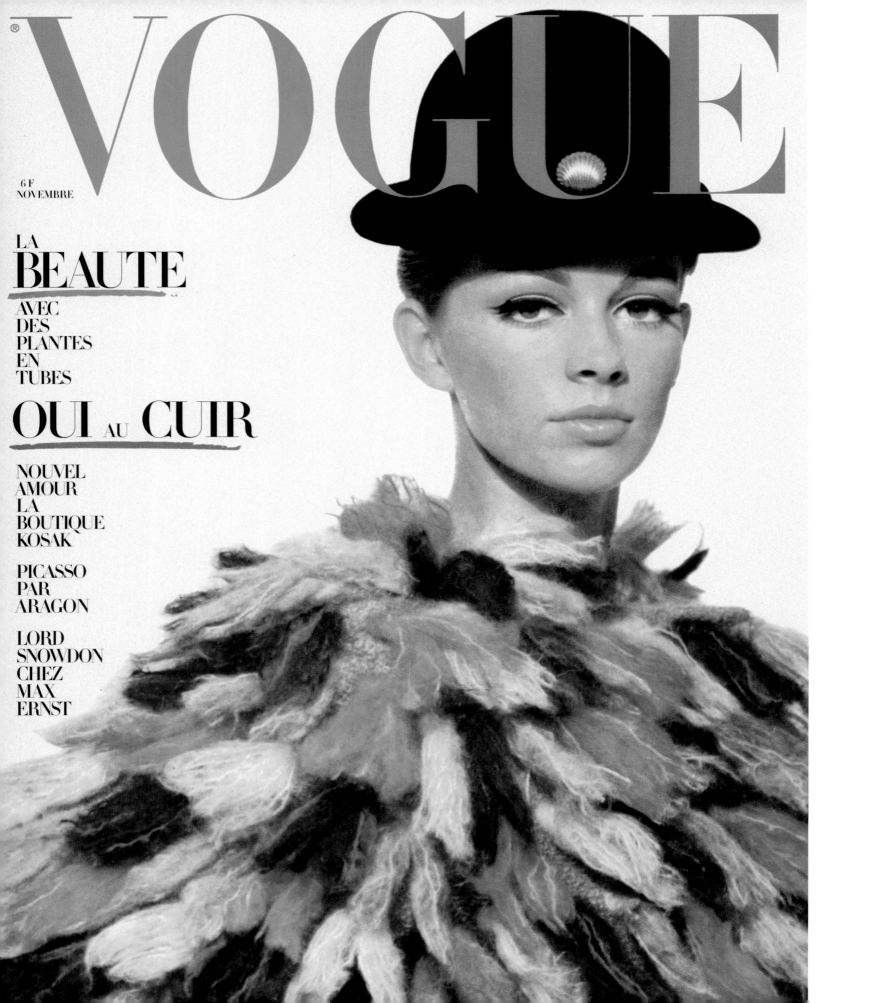

VOGUE

6 F
NOVEMBRE

LA
BEAUTE
AVEC
DES
PLANTES
EN
TUBES

OUI AU CUIR

NOUVEL
AMOUR
LA
BOUTIQUE
KOSAK

PICASSO
PAR
ARAGON

LORD
SNOWDON
CHEZ
MAX
ERNST

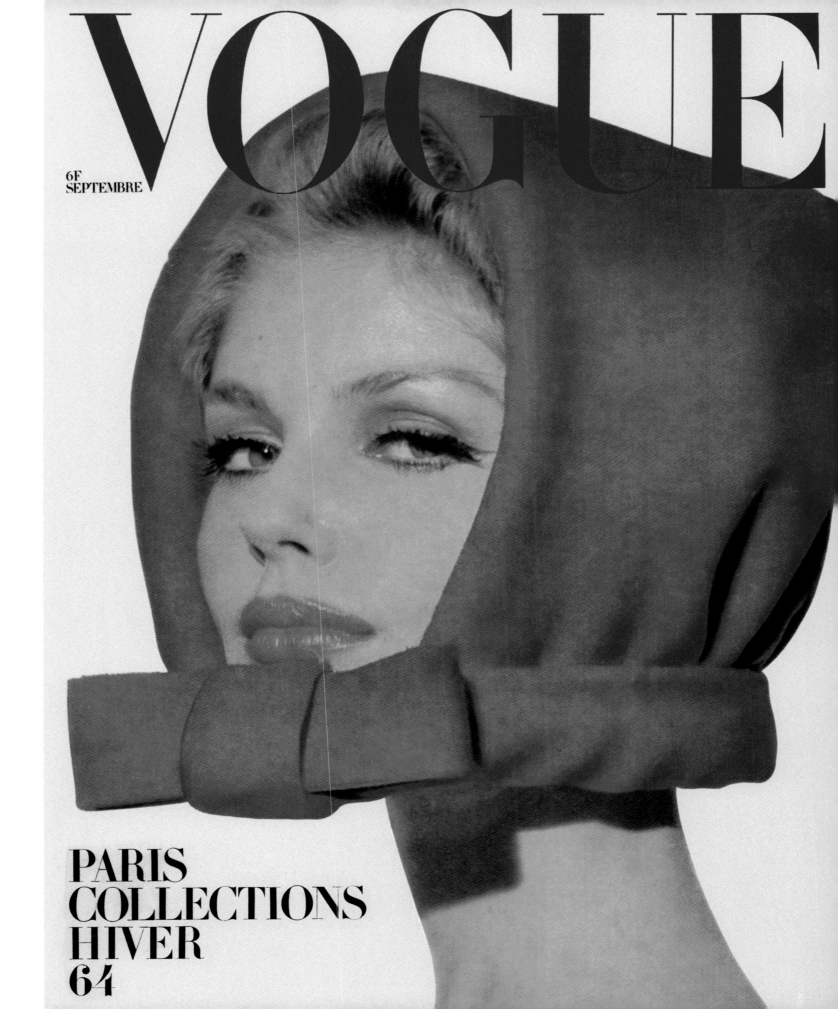

VOGUE

6F
SEPTEMBRE

PARIS
COLLECTIONS
HIVER
64

Christmas gems

'It was a gruelling prospect – composing the Christmas 1969 number of *Vogue* – but I admit I agreed to it without a qualm. For four reasons: I'm interested in fashion. *Vogue* has enormous potential, artistically and technically speaking. I love appearing confident and resourceful (although I'm neither). It will pay the upholsterer.'

— Françoise Sagan, *Vogue*, Christmas 1969

In 1969, Françoise Mohrt, *Vogue*'s Editor-in-Chief, first came up with the idea of producing a Christmas issue devoted to a celebrity. The writer Françoise Sagan (who had already contributed to the magazine) launched the formula. The cover photo, taken by Guy Bourdin, showed two models drenched in pearls and made up by Serge Lutens. 'One day, I received a call from a hairdresser out in the country,' Françoise Mohrt tells us. 'The man said to me: "Can you spare me a minute? I've designed some earrings." I replied: "What's so special about a pair of earrings?" He persisted, so I agreed to see him. He came into my office wearing a long frock coat and long black boots and it struck me that this man lived in a complete fantasy world. He told me, for example, that he could make false eyelashes from flies' wings. The man was Serge Lutens... I talked to Guy Bourdin about him and Guy was delighted to meet someone as mad as himself. He and Serge produced the Françoise Sagan cover. They wanted to illustrate the beauty of older women: this was the idea behind it...'[1]

With the exception of a ten-year period between 1993 and 2003, in which Christmas issues took a thematic focus (cinema, sciences, love, art, etc.), the annual Christmas celebrity issue has featured an extraordinarily prestigious series of guests (crucially, all unpaid), including Hitchcock, Chagall, Roman Polanski, Marlene Dietrich, Salvador Dalí, Miró, Fellini, David Hockney, Lauren Bacall, Orson Welles, Rostropovich, Kurosawa, Tàpies, the Dalai Lama and Nelson Mandela. The list is remarkable and provides an impressive series for the collector. 'The objective of the Christmas issue is not primarily commercial: the idea is that it should form part of a continuum and contribute to the enrichment of an existing library,' explains Olivier Lalanne, *Vogue*'s Assistant Editor since 2006, who commissioned the Catherine Deneuve, Sofia Coppola and Charlotte Gainsbourg issues. 'I'm often asked in relation to a particular person or subject: "But is it really *Vogue*?" The way I see it, the magazine is open to everything, but then it's a question of treatment.'

So, how does it work? What are the criteria for selecting a particular artist or celebrity? That depends on the editor's sensibilities, on circumstances and the particular mood of the moment. And, however fascinating the project may be, it requires the time and active participation of the guest celebrity. This is more than just an interview: it involves the insertion of another link in the production chain and launching into action with someone who is genuinely prepared to conduct the proceedings. 'People are usually very flattered to be asked, but they don't always realize how much work is involved,' says Lalanne. But when things are flowing as they should, the ease of communication is a journalist's dream: 'All Sofia Coppola had to do was lift the receiver and she was instantly connected with the whole of Hollywood!'

The success of these Christmas issues depends on the degree to which the special guest is prepared to be involved. Collaborating closely on one of these projects can be a memorable experience – working, for example, with Hitchcock, bedridden following heart surgery and receiving the team in his English manor house where the shadows had an uncannily Hitchcockian feel, or with Charlotte Gainsbourg as she told the story of every nook and cranny of the paternal temple in rue de Verneuil, or with the painter Tàpies, communicating exclusively through the medium of his brushes and canvases…

Certain issues have acquired an almost mythical dimension. This is the case with the 1989 issue produced in conjunction with the cellist Mstislav Rostropovich. Colombe Pringle, who edited the magazine between 1986 and 1994, recalls the particularly awkward circumstances surrounding its completion. 'We had arranged to meet at Rostropovich's house, in Paris, so that we could finalize the layouts. Rostropovich wasn't there. We waited and finally we learned that he had gone off to Berlin in a mad hurry. The Wall had just come down, and he wanted to be a part of it. Everyone can remember those scenes of Rostropovich mucking about in the crowd, in front of a section of the ruined wall. They've become legendary. We couldn't leave that out, obviously, in an issue that was devoted to him. And we didn't have the time to go to Berlin. So our Art Director used some of the TV images, which added a really moving sense of immediacy.' The cover itself was risky: by opting for a drawing by Sempé (which was not easy to see from a distance), rather than a portrait of the musician, the editors were taking a chance on what might appeal to a collector rather than making an obvious commercial choice.

Another legendary issue, which commands increasingly high prices today, was the 1992 edition dedicated to the Dalai Lama. Colombe Pringle comments: 'It was a big year for Madonna. Everyone was talking about her. But it was also the aftermath of the Gulf War. A lot of questions were being asked. Richard Gere announced that he was a Buddhist. There was a certain something in the air, and I trusted it. Via a series of contacts, we succeeded in meeting the Dalai Lama in April in Salzburg, where he granted us a quarter-of-an-hour interview. I'd taken along some copies of *Vogue* and I gave him a quick explanation. He looked me in the eyes and simply said: "Come and see me in Dharamsala with a hundred questions." "When?" I asked. "September," he replied. I thanked him and we set to work. We spent several months calling on different specialists and finally came up with a hundred questions, spiritual, historical, cultural, social, aesthetic, all sorts… Then we travelled as planned – a team of just six of us – to see him in his monastery. We stayed in his mother's old house and he received us every morning for a week, answering all our questions and commenting on the photos and the layouts. At the end of our stay, I asked him why he'd stipulated a hundred questions. He replied: "It was just a joke!" The cover for that issue is a publicity image, an album sleeve carrying a picture of him which we found in a small shop in Dharamsala…' The magazine sold out very quickly. Some people liked it, others wondered what the theme had to do with a women's magazine. 'We weren't looking for legitimacy, and I was criticized for that,' says Pringle. 'But that is part of what makes *Vogue* such an absolute luxury, so elitist – that it can do something completely gratuitous and see it through… And anyway our advertisers were often rather pleased to appear in these editions.'

Following the Dalai Lama coup, Pringle wanted to 'strike' as hard again and she persuaded Nelson Mandela to cooperate. The issue appeared just as Mandela was awarded the Nobel Peace Prize and was preparing to take over the South African presidency. These encounters with history clearly gave *Vogue*'s Christmas issues an additional impact and proved that these special issues were above all the fruit of genuine journalistic effort, of an ability to capture a contemporary mood and identify a niche, reflect the times and stand by editorial decisions. When in 2005, under the direction of Carine Roitfeld, *Vogue* offered a very different sort of celebrity – Kate Moss – the opportunity to feature in the Christmas issue, the choice may have seemed at first rather obvious. But in the autumn, just as work was about to begin on the issue, due out in December, the supermodel disappeared from circulation to undertake a programme for drug rehabilitation. She was caught up in a cocaine scandal, her private life was in disarray, and many of the big fashion houses that used her image swiftly abandoned her. *Vogue*, however, chose to support Moss in defiance of negative public opinion, and despite all the difficulties of producing a magazine when its guest of honour was absent, the issue still came out on time. 'The media storm that greeted her on her return never once weakened [our] resolve. The supermodel of the century may not be a model person, but she is still, for women and designers alike, the most inspiring of muses,' we read in the magazine's editorial. Christmas *Vogue* that year was a success.

1 In an interview conducted in 1995 by Susan Train.

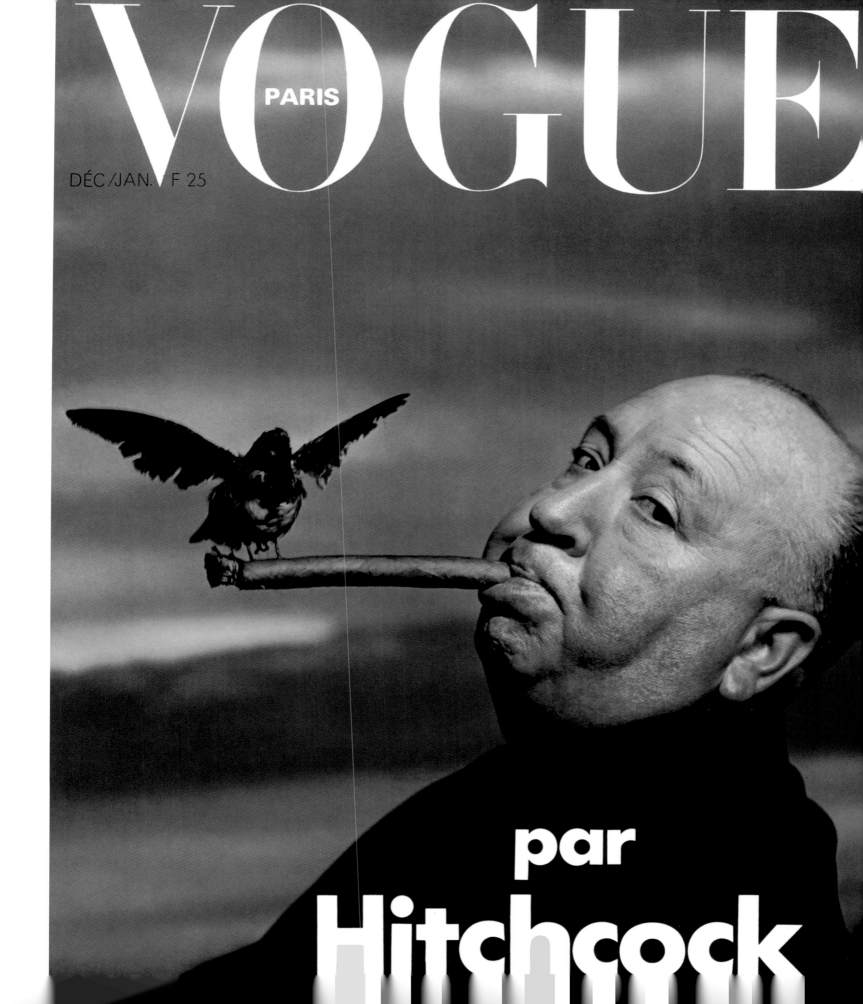

VOGUE
PARIS

DÉC./JAN. F 25

par
Hitchcock

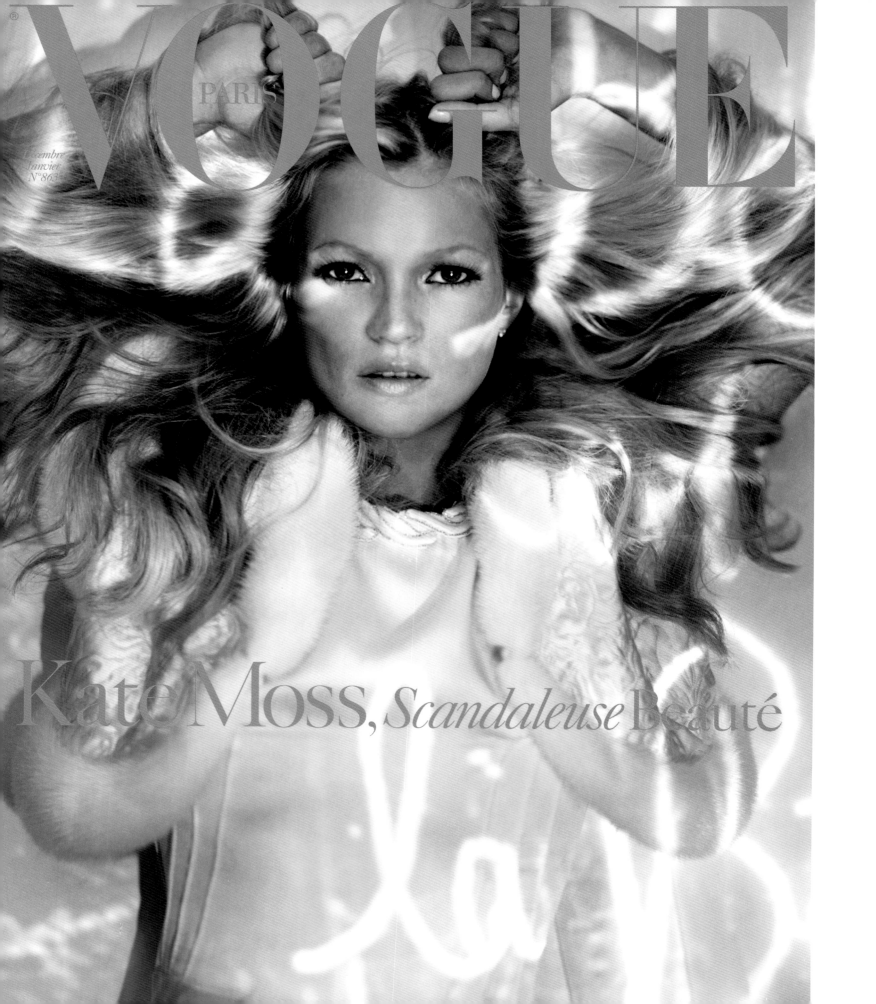

VOGUE

PARIS

Décembre
Janvier
N° 863

Kate Moss, *Scandaleuse Beauté*

VOGUE

PARIS

Décembre
Janvier

Kate Moss, *Scandaleuse* Beauté

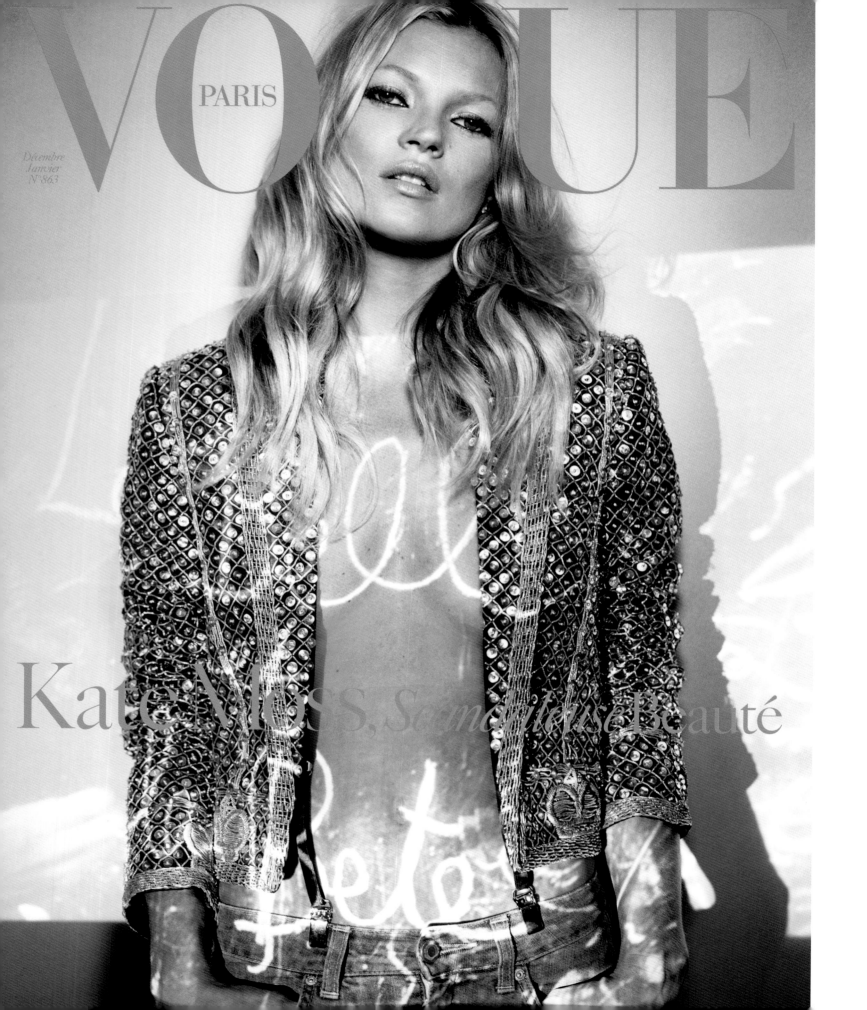

VOGUE

PARIS

Décembre
Janvier
N°863

Kate Moss, Scandaleuse Beauté

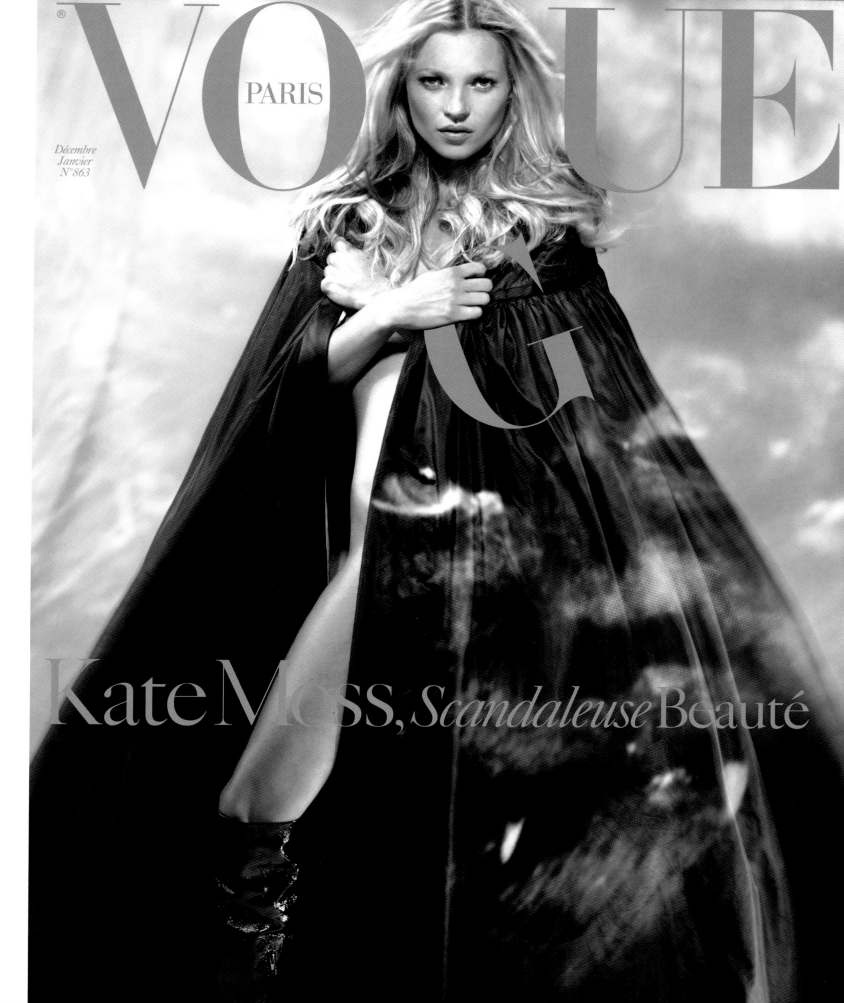

VOGUE

PARIS

Décembre
Janvier
N° 863

Kate Moss, *Scandaleuse Beauté*

VOGUE

PARIS

DÉC./JAN.   F 40

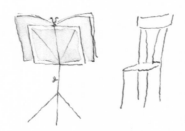

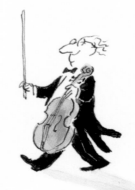

sempé

PAR

ROSTROPOVICH

PREVIOUS PAGES
December 2005
by Kate Moss
Craig McDean
Couturiers:
p. 108 Valentino Couture
p. 109 Dior Homme by Hedi Slimane
and Armani
p. 110 Dior Homme by Hedi Slimane
p. 111 Givenchy Haute Couture

OPPOSITE
December 1989
by Rostropovich
Sempé

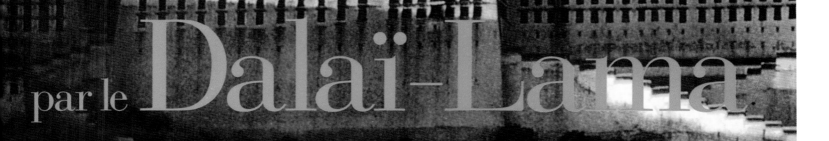

VOGUE
PARIS

DÉC./JAN.   F.40

par le Dalaï-Lama

VOGUE

PARIS

DEC./JAN. F 40

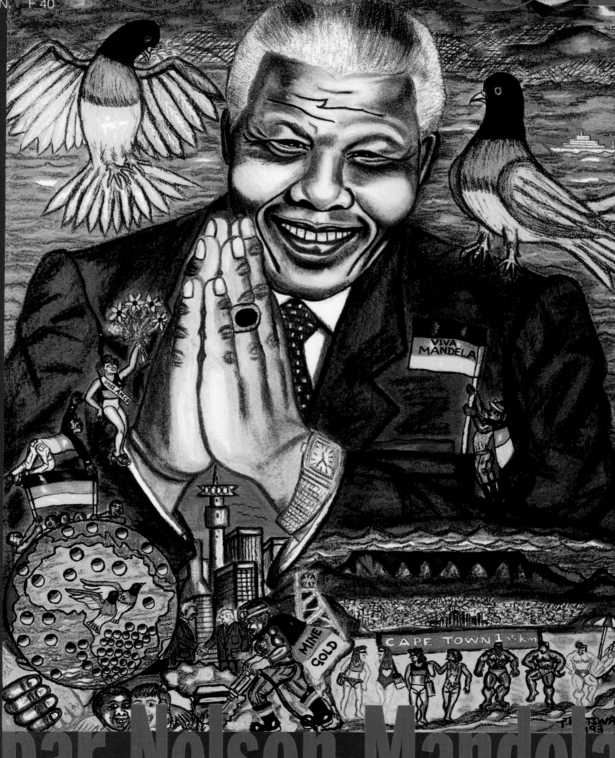

par Nelson Mandela

VOGUE

PARIS

DÉC./JAN. F 30

PAR

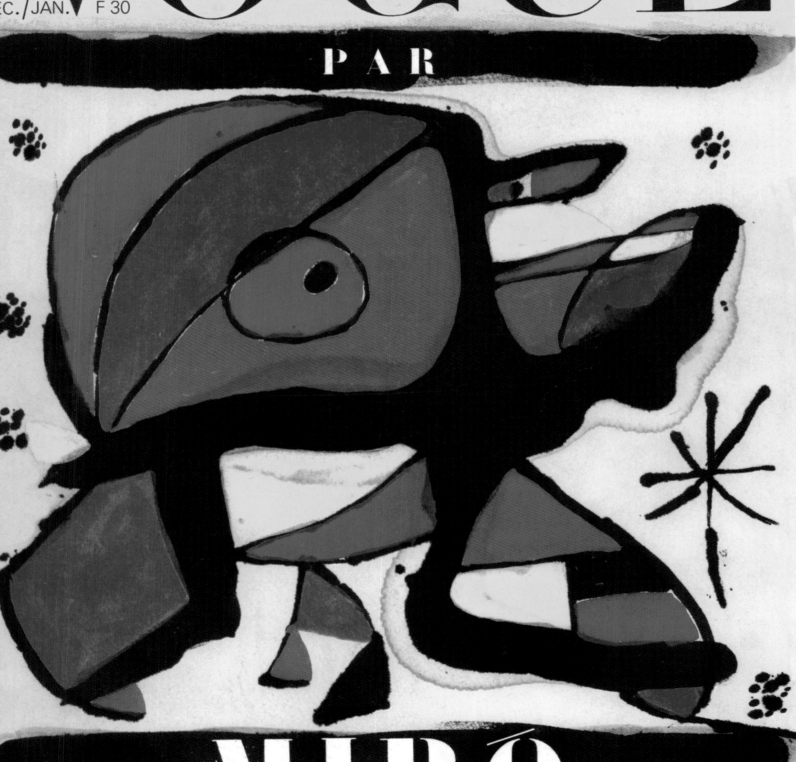

MIRÓ

VOGUE

PARIS

DÉC
JAN

F 40

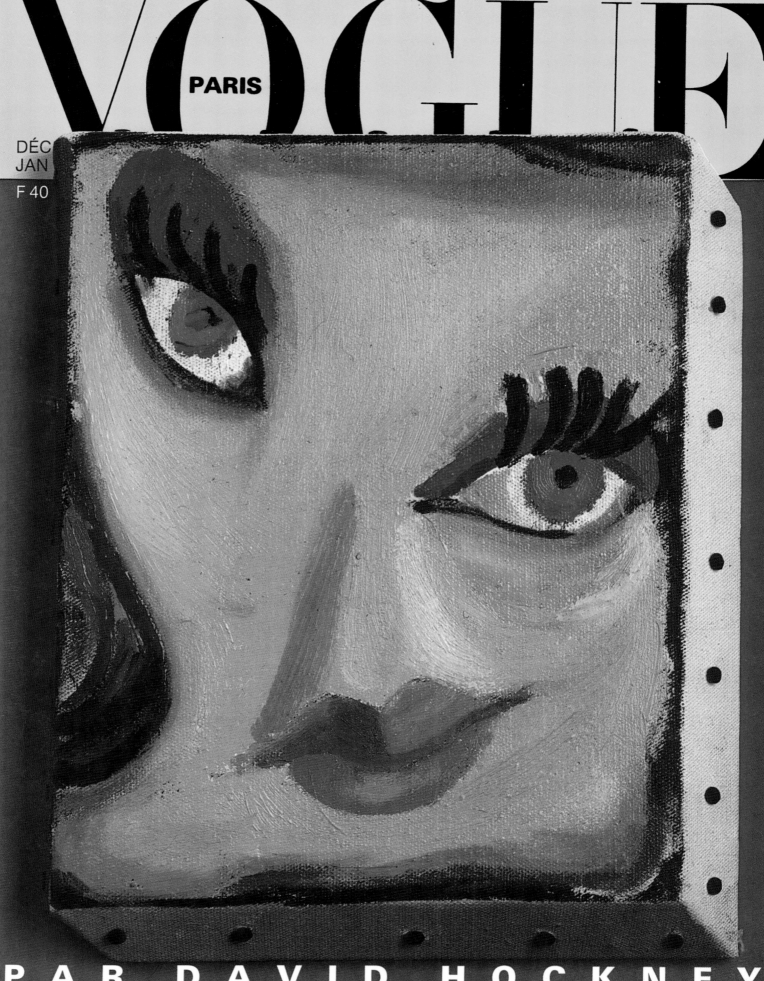

PAR DAVID HOCKNEY

PREVIOUS PAGES
December 1992
by the Dalai Lama
Artist unknown

December 1993
by Nelson Mandela
Tommy Mostwai

December 1979
by Joan Miró

December 1985
by David Hockney

OPPOSITE
December 1983
by Caroline of Monaco
Andy Warhol

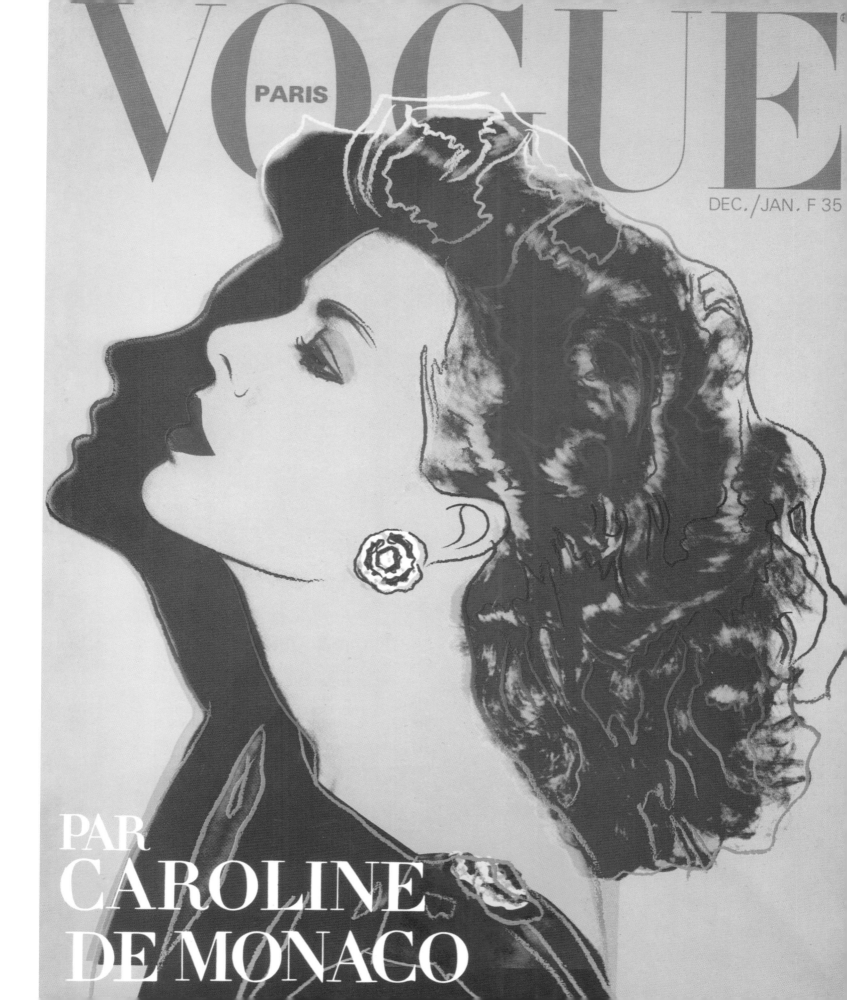

VOGUE

PARIS

DEC./JAN. F 35

PAR
CAROLINE
DE MONACO

VOGUE

PARIS

Décembre
Janvier
N° 873

NOËL
DANS LA
PEAU DE
John Galliano
SPECIAL GUEST
DREW
BARRYMORE.

VOGUE
PARIS

Décembre
Janvier
N° 873

NOËL
DANS LA
PEAU DE
John Galliano
SPECIAL GUEST
DREW
BARRYMORE.

VOGUE

PARIS

DÉC .
JAN . F 25

NUMÉRO DU CINQUANTENAIRE
1921/1971 RÉALISÉ PAR
SALVADOR
DALI

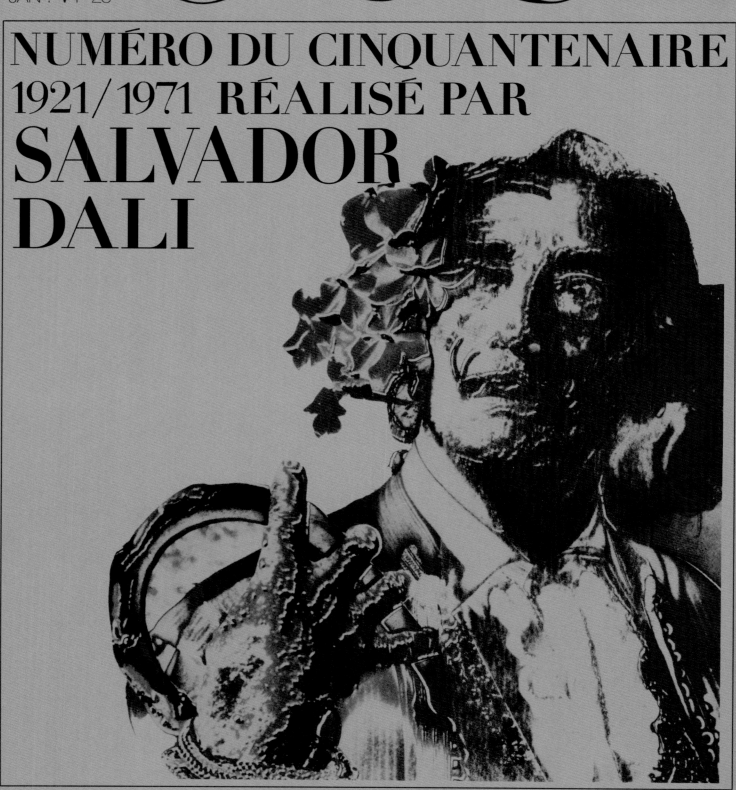

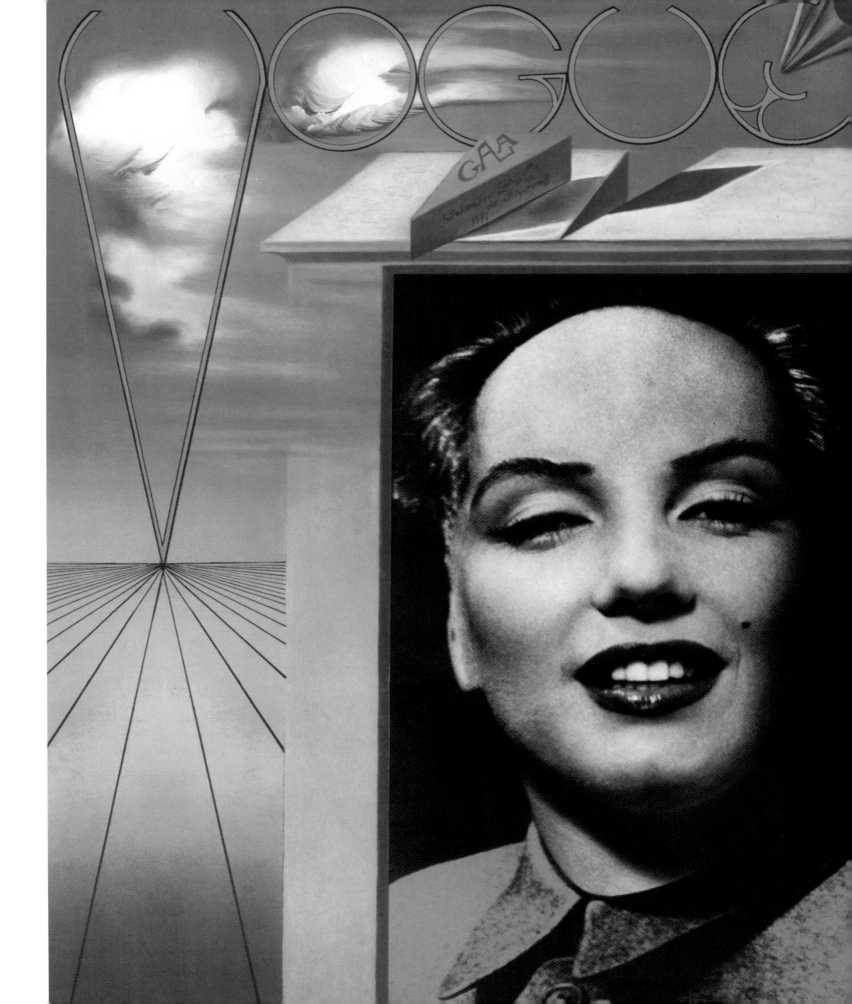

PREVIOUS PAGES
December 2006
by John Galliano
Nick Knight
Model Drew Barrymore
Couturiers:
p. 120 John Galliano
p. 121 Dior Haute Couture
by John Galliano

December 1971
by Salvador Dalí
p. 123 photo of Marilyn Monroe
Philippe Halsman

OPPOSITE
December 2004
by Sofia Coppola
Mario Testino
Couturier Marc Jacobs

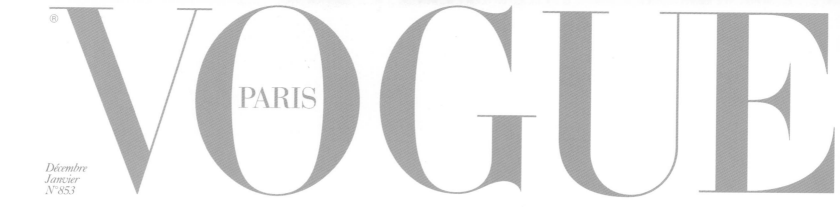

VOGUE PARIS

Décembre
Janvier
N° 853

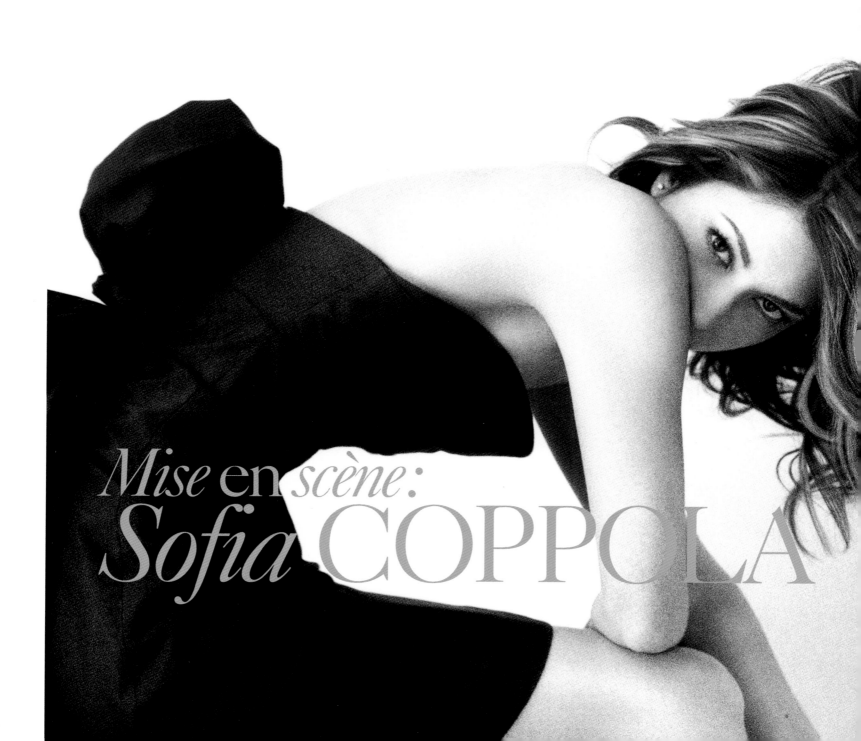

Mise en scène :
Sofia COPPOLA

VOGUE

PARIS

DÉC./JAN. F 30

PAR

Marc Chagall

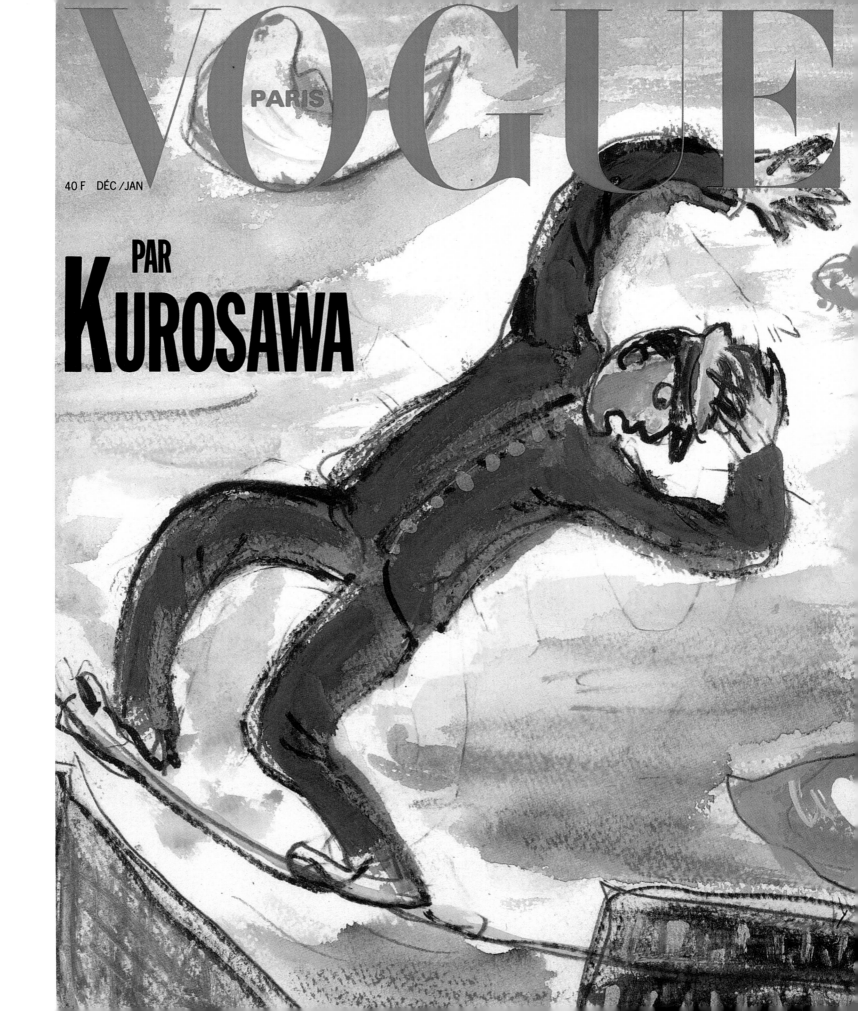

VOGUE

PARIS

40 F   DÉC /JAN

PAR KUROSAWA

VOGUE

PARIS

Décembre
Janvier
N° 843

par Catherine
DENEUVE

Paris

'Paris makes more than the law, she makes fashion.'
— Victor Hugo, *Les Misérables*

It was not until 1968 that the covers of French *Vogue* carried any mention of Paris. But from then on, this 'Paris' was routinely associated with the *Vogue* logo, whose graphics have stayed exactly the same since 1953. These decisions emanated from the Condé Nast company's desire to give the title of the magazine greater impact and to raise it to the level of an international brand name, which consequently needed to be readily identifiable. Following the American, English and French editions, the idea was to develop other editions of *Vogue* (there are some fifteen worldwide today), each of them enjoying the benefit of association with the same famous name while retaining its distinctness by being rooted in the life and customs of a particular country.

Vogue France had of course long focused its attention on the artistic and cultural life of the capital. In March 1940, the city had featured on one of *Vogue*'s last pre-Occupation covers, in the form of a very Parisian hat seen in close-up, with two soldiers, marching side by side, advancing in the background. With the return of peacetime, Paris in the sunshine under cloudless skies was splashed across the magazine's front covers. In the aftermath of the Liberation, the city become one of the main strands of the magazine, regularly referenced on the front cover: illustrations and photos invoked the city, in particular through images of its most famous monuments, symbols that were immediately recognizable. Léone Friedrich, a shorthand typist who joined the magazine in 1927, recalls the first issue to appear after the war, in the winter of 1945–46: 'It was an illustration of the Place de la Concorde by the artist Nerebriarova, dominated by a blue sky and white clouds. This cover was originally intended for the autumn issue, September 1939. But we didn't get it out then and it ended up being used for the first post-war issue.'[1]

A great many questions were being asked in the post-war period, as Edmonde Charles-Roux, who joined the magazine in 1947, recounts: 'Michel de Brunhoff was the Editor-in-Chief and working alongside him was his brother-in-law, Lucien Vogel, who had very close links with the Condé Nast magazines and was well in with the editorial staff. There was a constant dialogue going on between Michel and Vogel and a lot of questions were being asked, generally, with regard to the re-launch of *Vogue* after the Liberation. You have to remember that no one knew at that time whether haute couture would actually recover, and in particular whether it would ever regain its original standing. There was no Maison Dior yet, and neither Schiaparelli nor Rochas nor Chanel had reopened. As for the society columns, one of the backbones of the magazine, which never missed a ball or a wedding or a reception, the same air of uncertainty hung over them, due to the number of families in mourning and the number of châteaux that had been destroyed. I remember one particular weekend in the country, at the Vogels' house: after dinner, Lucien, who was a real press wizard, and had created the magazine *Vu*, the true forerunner of *Match*, said: "We can't recreate the pre-war *Vogue*. What we need to do now is develop a truly Parisian magazine that couldn't be dreamed up in Rome or London or New York. We need a real window on Paris..."'[2]

If Lucien Vogel launched the idea, Michel de Brunhoff was the ideal person to put it into practice. He was no socialite, but enjoyed the good life and was intimately connected with some of the great artistic and literary figures of the day – designers, painters, sculptors, novelists and playwrights including the likes of Jouvet, Cocteau, Picasso, Chagall, Colette and Bérard, whom he saw on a daily basis, at cafés and bars and for Sunday outings in the country. Brunhoff was more of an editor than a journalist and his talent for page design and flair for nosing out and collaborating with the best artists, illustrators and photographers made him a key actor on the Paris arts stage.

In 1947, a new column began appearing in the magazine, signed by André Ostier. 'La vie à Paris' – 'Paris Life' – reflected the cultural vitality of the capital, and in its first edition mention was made of André Malraux, Gérard Philippe, Simone de

Beauvoir, Louis Aragon, Roland Petit and Albert Camus. Other columns, appearing in parallel in the American and English editions, focused on contemporary events in New York and London, highlighting the distinctive nature of each of these cities.

Michel de Brunhoff put particular emphasis on Paris's theatrical performances and shows, where the photographic opportunities were especially exciting, and he hired Edmonde Charles-Roux to go to every performance throughout the capital. 'We have the best stage designers in the world, there's no denying,' he told her, and from now on a great many pages were devoted to theatre sets, such as those designed by Christian Bérard for Louis Jouvet, by André Derain and Max Ernst for Roland Petit, and Jean Carzou for the Opéra de Paris. Painters brought their sketches to the magazine, and *Vogue* was an address where members of the art world regularly crossed paths. They were soon to be followed by writers, with the introduction of a literary column by Edmonde Charles-Roux, appointed Editor-in-Chief in 1954. François Mauriac, Simone de Beauvoir, Françoise Giroud and later Marguerite Duras, Jean Genet and Françoise Sagan all wrote for *Vogue* – though this unconventional development did not come about without some controversy at the magazine, especially in the publicity department, where the fear was that it might put off the advertisers. Edmonde Charles-Roux recalls arguing that: 'just because a woman is rich doesn't mean she's an idiot', an attitude in which she was supported by Philippe de Croisset, then Director General of Condé Nast France, who commented: 'The purchasing power is in the hands of wealthy women. Why would they not buy books for themselves?'

The covers featuring the capital announced the magazine's new identity, based on a distinctive cultural and artistic flair. They were soon also celebrating the renewed vigour of haute couture, which, from 1947, thanks in particular to Christian Dior's 'New Look', had recovered its pre-eminence and its influence across the globe. Above all the magazine sought to stand out from other publications by exploiting whatever riches were at hand. Hence, for example, the contract signed by Michel de Brunhoff in 1950 with the photographer Robert Doisneau, whose photographs captured the essence of Paris better than any other. Also the close collaborations with Christian Bérard and Gruau, whose fashion illustrations were synonymous with Parisian tastes, and also a great many covers signed by William Klein, American by birth, Parisian by adoption and inclination.

1 In an interview conducted by Susan Train in 1995.

2 *Idem*

November 1930
Georges Lepape

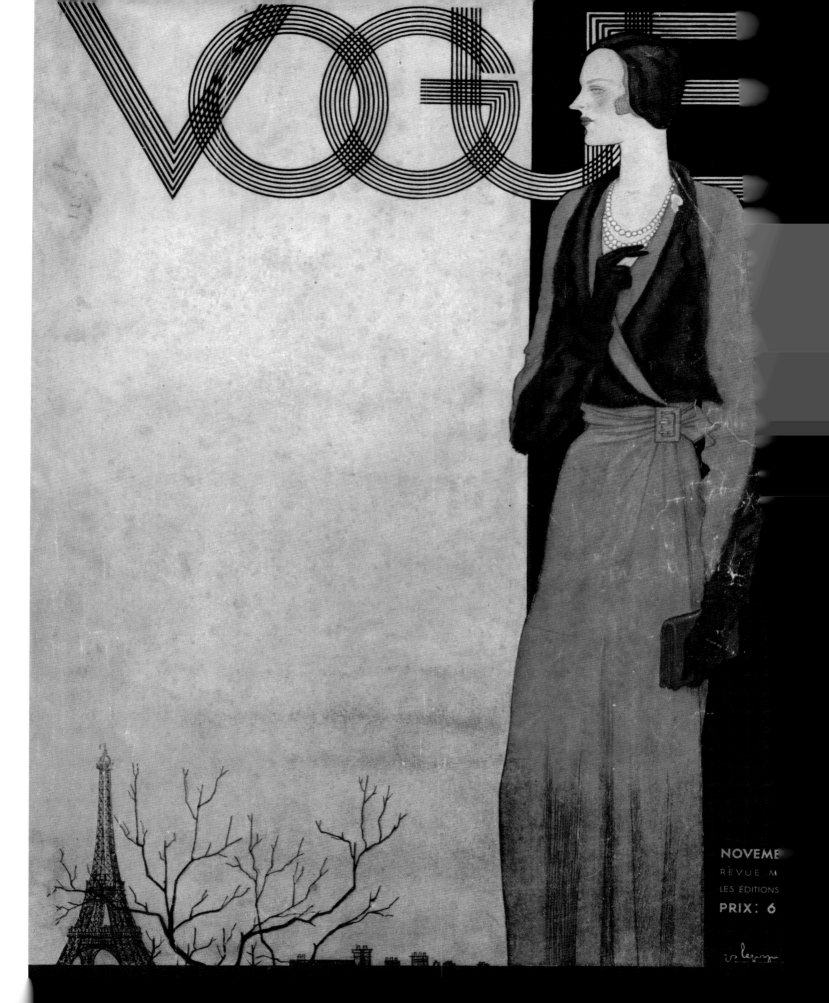

VOGUE

NOVEMBE

RÈVUE M

LES ÉDITIONS

PRIX: 6

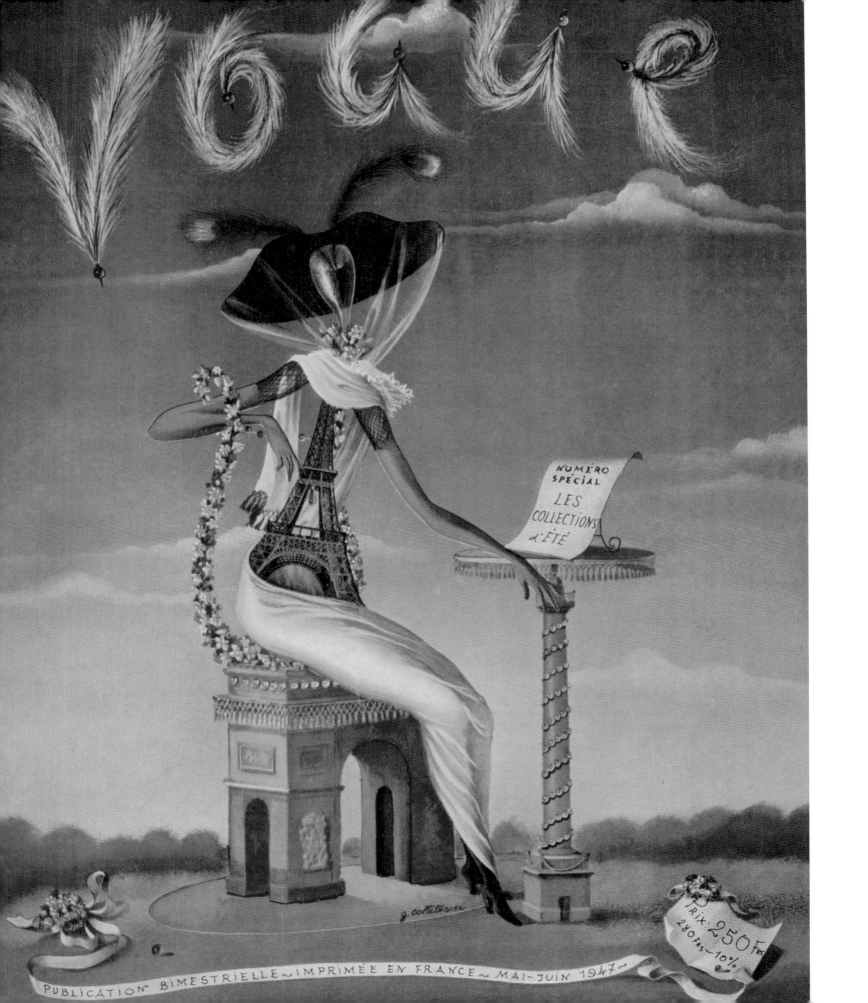

NUMÉRO
SPÉCIAL
LES
COLLECTIONS
d'ÉTÉ

PUBLICATION BIMESTRIELLE ~ IMPRIMÉE EN FRANCE ~ MAI-JUIN 1947 ~

Prix: 250 Frs
280 frs — 10%

VOGUE

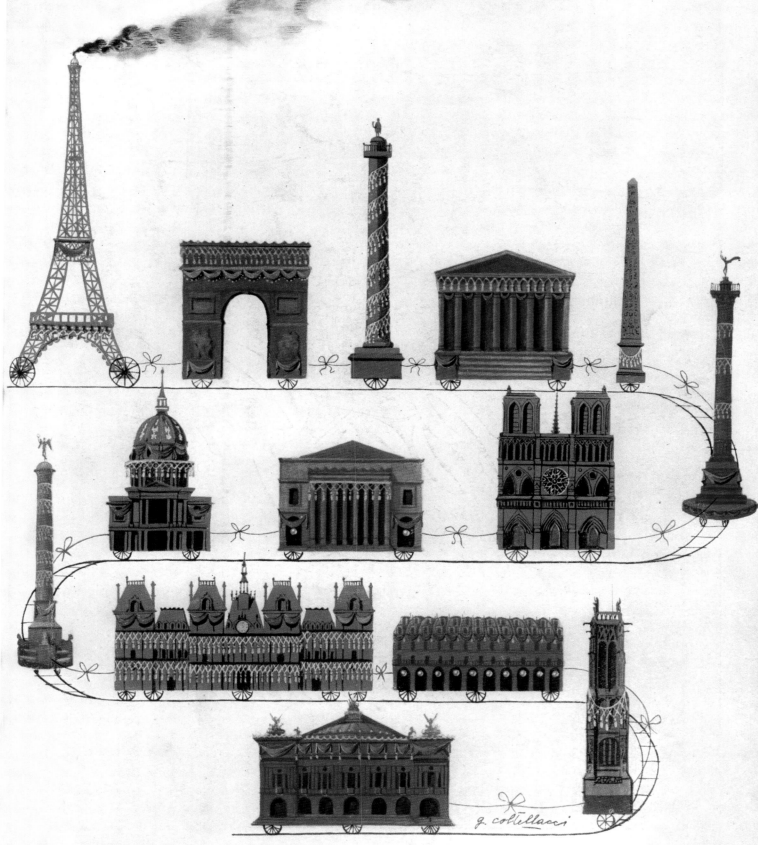

g. coltellacci

CHAPEAUX · FOURRURES · PREMIERS MODÈLES D'AUTOMNE

SEPTEMBRE 1949 · REVUE MENSUELLE IMPRIMÉE EN FRANCE · PRIX : 350 FRS.

VOGUE

PARIS A 2.000 ANS • LES COLLECTIONS DE PLEIN ÉTÉ

JUIN 1951 • REVUE MENSUELLE IMPRIMÉE EN FRANCE • 500 FRANCS

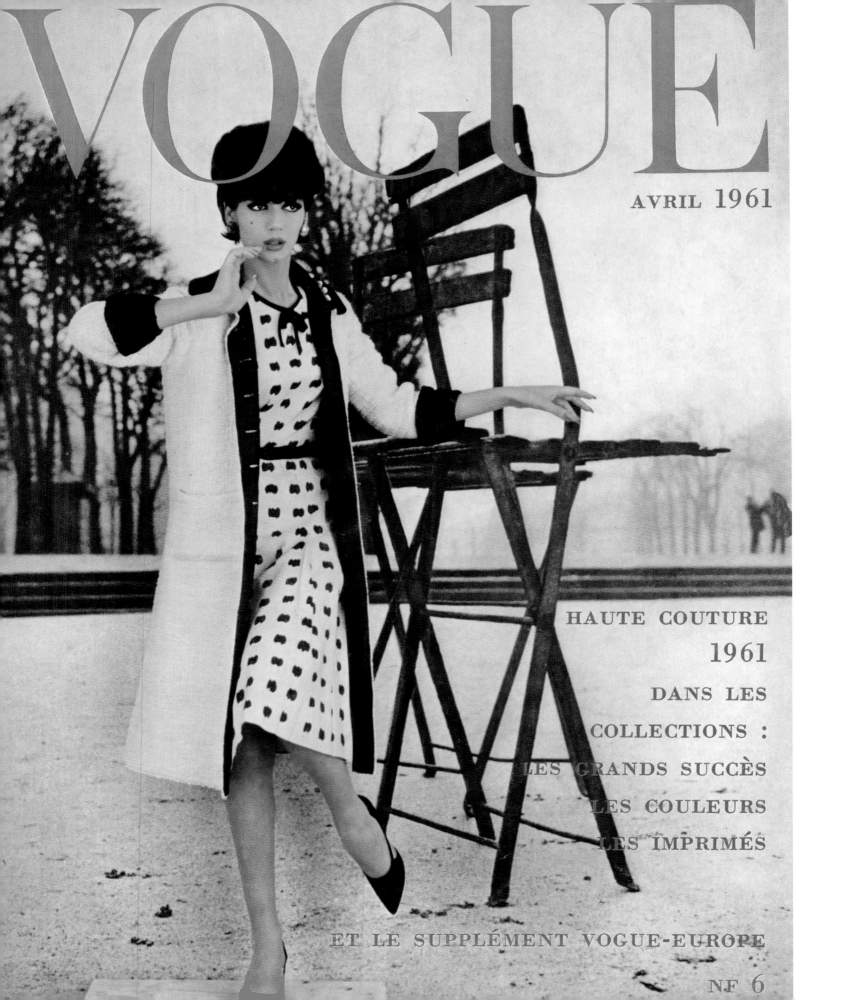

VOGUE

AVRIL 1961

HAUTE COUTURE

1961

DANS LES

COLLECTIONS :

LES GRANDS SUCCÈS

LES COULEURS

LES IMPRIMÉS

ET LE SUPPLÉMENT VOGUE-EUROPE

NF 6

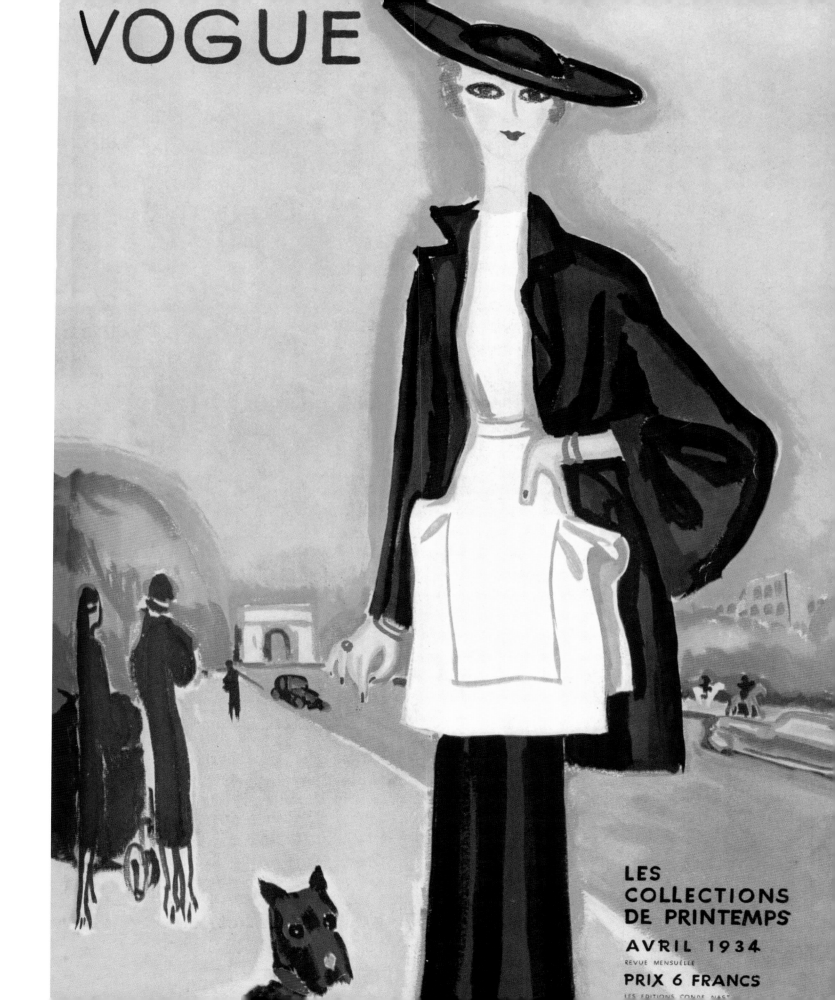

VOGUE

LES
COLLECTIONS
DE PRINTEMPS
AVRIL 1934
REVUE MENSUELLE
PRIX 6 FRANCS
LES ÉDITIONS CONDÉ NAST

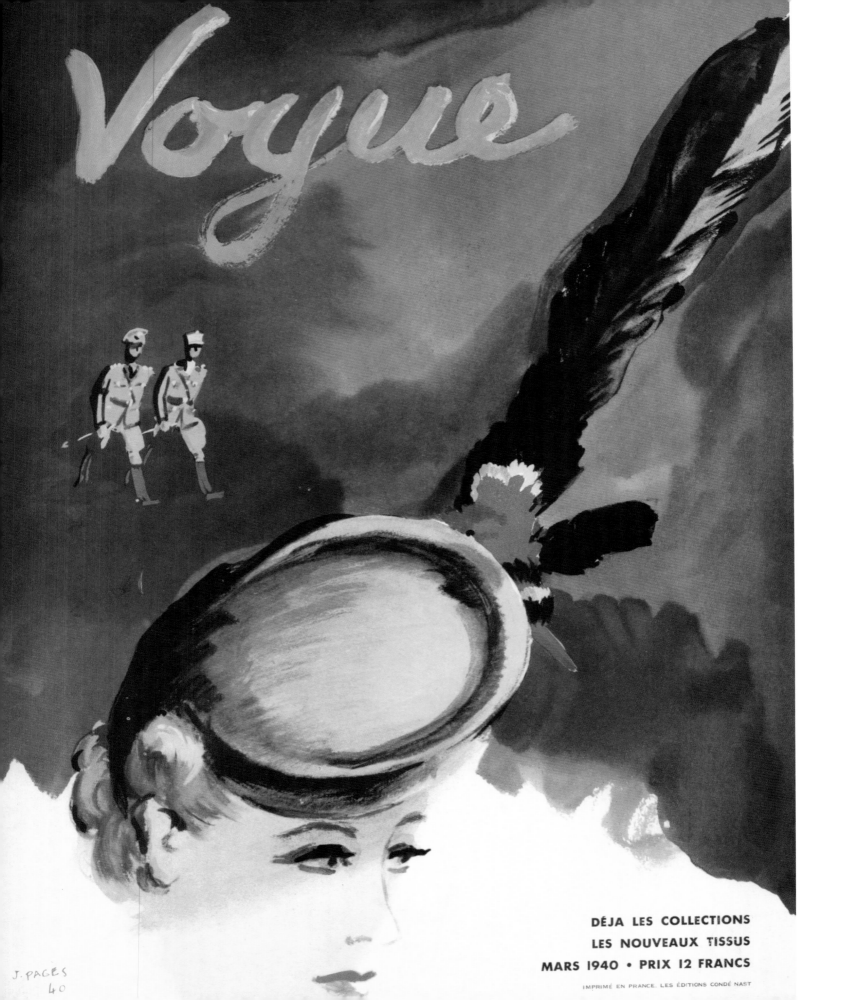

Vogue

DÉJA LES COLLECTIONS

LES NOUVEAUX TISSUS

MARS 1940 • PRIX 12 FRANCS

IMPRIMÉ EN FRANCE. LES ÉDITIONS CONDÉ NAST

J. PAGÈS
40

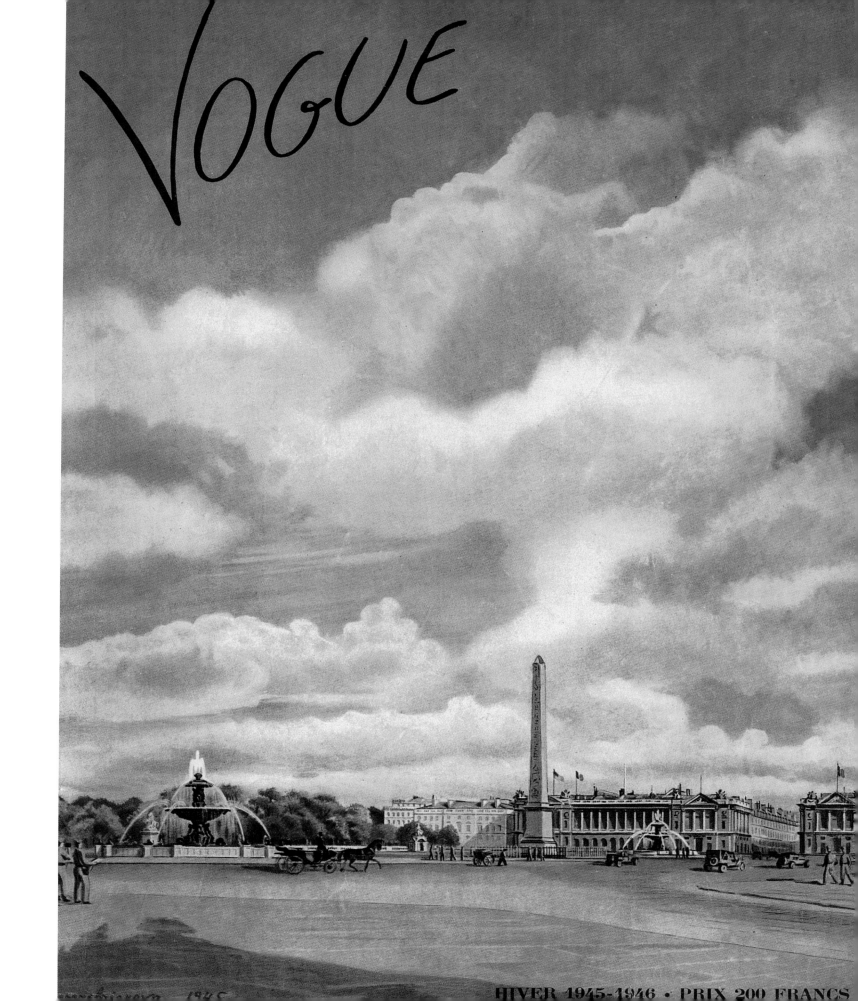

VOGUE

HIVER 1945-1946 • PRIX 200 FRANCS

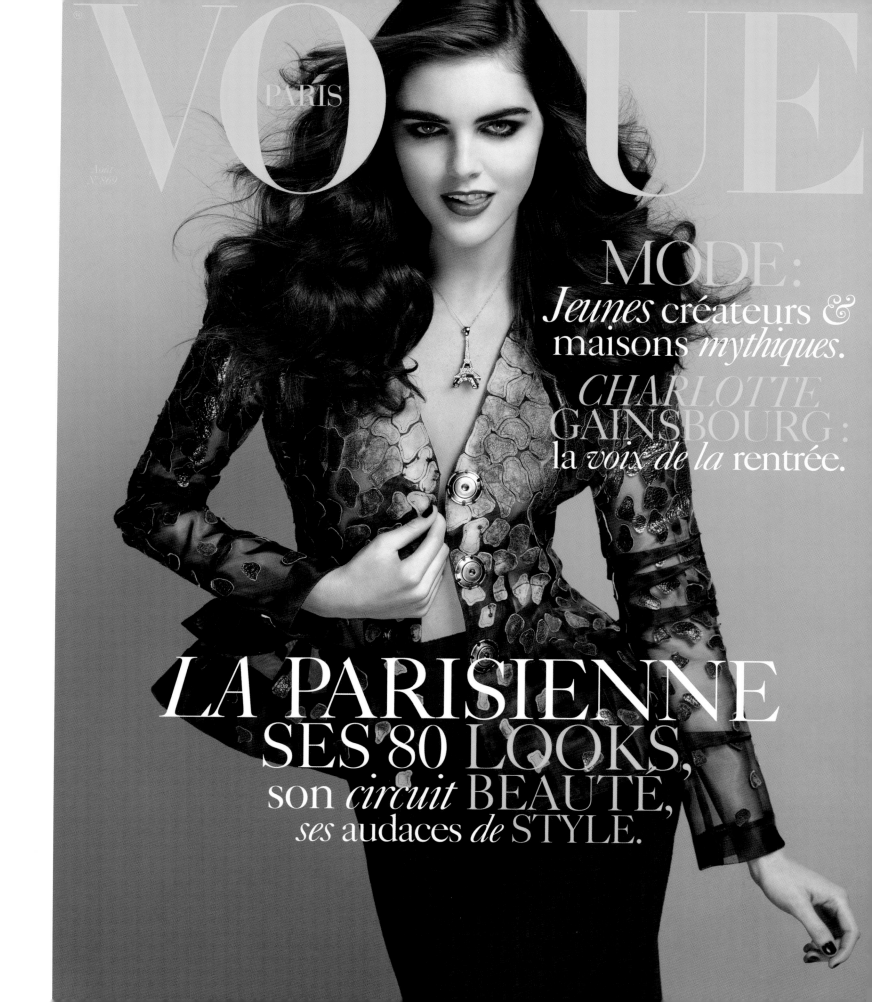

VOGUE

PARIS

Août
N° 869

MODE:
Jeunes créateurs &
maisons *mythiques*.

CHARLOTTE
GAINSBOURG:
la *voix de la* rentrée.

LA PARISIENNE
SES 80 LOOKS,
son *circuit* BEAUTÉ,
ses audaces *de* STYLE.

Star system

'The quintessential French woman in the eyes of the world, Catherine Deneuve is passionate, a free spirit, and an actress with an impressive list of film credits to her name. Where she was concerned, the editorial staff were unanimous.'
— Carine Roitfeld, *Vogue*, Christmas 2003

'She's eighteen years old, she's gorgeous, she's just had her first major success with *Les Parisiennes*, and she's agreed to pose for us.' It was April 1962 and the young woman in question was Catherine Deneuve, appearing for the first time on *Vogue*'s front cover. There was, however, no mention of her name, which only appeared as part of the caption to Helmut Newton's photo inside the magazine.

This was a 'first' that was significant in more ways than one. For more than forty years, Catherine Deneuve has held the record (by a wide margin) for the number of *Vogue* covers on which she has featured: the figure stands at sixteen today, the last taken by Mario Testino for the Christmas 2003 edition devoted to her. More than any other celebrity, Deneuve seems to embody the true essence of *Vogue*, as we are reminded by the editorial for that special issue: 'The quintessential French woman in the eyes of the world, Catherine Deneuve is passionate, a free spirit, and an actress with an impressive list of film credits to her name. Where she was concerned, the editorial staff were unanimous.' In the opinion of the photographers, led by Guy

Bourdin, who had a reputation for being hard on his models, she was also a great professional, ready to bow to the demands of the camera – which, in the 1960s, were a great deal more onerous than they are today. Deneuve thus met all of *Vogue*'s requirements, including those of class and elegance, an elegance that has always been associated with the man who dressed her, her friend the couturier Yves Saint Laurent.

Vogue has never set out to be a 'people' magazine. On the contrary, it has always assumed the role of arbiter and dictator of fashion, and it is this orientation that the April 1962 cover also highlights. Deneuve was still relatively unknown: she was only to burst into the limelight two years later in Jacques Demy's *Les Parapluies de Cherbourg* ('The Umbrellas of Cherbourg'), which won the 1964 Palme d'Or at Cannes. Not only did her name not appear beside the image (it would be more than ten years and several covers later before that happened); there was no interview with her inside the magazine. Supermodels did not yet exist, and so images of young actresses were used to bring a touch of glamour to the magazine. During the 1960s and 1970s, they succeeded one another in the fashion pages or on the front covers of *Vogue* at a steady rate. Whether just starting out in their career or at the height of their fame, these women were selected because they corresponded to the criteria of chic and style that were *Vogue*'s aspiration and rallying cry. These fresh young leading ladies were the new icons of the '*Vogue* touch': Marthe Keller, Geraldine Chaplin, Anny Duperey, Marisa Berenson, Charlotte Rampling, Brigitte Bardot, Jane Birkin, Dani, Ursula Andress, Marie Laforêt, Sylvie Vartan, Dominique Sanda, Sydne Rome, Jacqueline Bisset, Dayle Haddon and Margaux Hemingway succeeded one another and often featured together, in the fashion pages and in close-up on the cover, although there were never more than a couple of lines regarding their private or professional lives. In contrast with the aristocratic icons of the 1930s – society women whose photographs placed them on a pedestal, firmly out of reach – these women, many of them popular and French, embodied a familiar, reassuring type of beauty and presented an image with which the reader could readily identify. Neither remote goddess nor girl next door, they were 'accessible stars', whose physical appearance was what primarily interested *Vogue*. But, as always, there were exceptions. When a romantic image of the American actress Audrey Hepburn appeared on the cover of *Vogue* in May 1963, it was actually as a way of celebrating Hubert de Givenchy, one of the great names of French couture. Hepburn was a major player on the Hollywood scene and a star of international standing, who was about to film George Cukor's *My Fair Lady* (with costumes by the photographer and designer Cecil Beaton, a regular contributor to *Vogue*). For ten years, she had been Givenchy's muse and her name features large alongside the cover photo, while a substantial section of the magazine is devoted to her comments regarding the couturier's talent and his collections: it was fashion that justified this star's appearance, and not vice versa.

This approach continued through the latter half of the 1980s and into the 1990s: when, for example, Stephanie and Caroline of Monaco appeared on the cover in 1986 and 1988 respectively, it was a way of reconnecting with the magazine's original identity while also remaining 'in the moment'. The two princesses, both pictured in haughty poses, were bona fide royalty and members of the jet set, as well as possessing a youth and beauty that were the perfect representation of their age. One of them was putting her name to clothes and songs, while the other was a close friend of Karl Lagerfeld, among others, and a patron of the arts. They perfectly embodied the triumphant glamour of the 1980s, while simultaneously meeting all the requirements of the *Vogue* icon: aristocratic, cosmopolitan, confidently stylish and actively feminine. Who could the cover feature after that? The challenge was laid down: with the development of the media and intensification of publicity campaigns of all kinds, celebrities were making ever more frequent appearances in the press. If *Vogue* was to continue to stand out, it had to look further afield. The focus shifted away from everyday stars to the myth-makers – Madonna, the ultimate idol; Isabelle Adjani, the personification of mystery; Juliette Binoche, the petite French woman sought by the great... The choices were restricted, so much so that between 1996 and 2003 not a single star appeared on a *Vogue* cover.

In August of 2003, Sophie Marceau ushered in a new era. Olivier Lalanne, *Vogue*'s Assistant Editor, recalls that 'since the year 2000, anyone can "treat" themselves to a star, so *Vogue* has adopted the principle of providing a completely new emphasis, extricating itself from the promotional rut and creating added value, doing something surprising'. The August 2003 issue is particularly significant in this regard. The cover carries the headline 'Marceau, la vérité' ('Marceau, the truth'). The actress was not promoting any particular film at the time, but nevertheless agreed to be the subject of an intimate portrait that pulled no punches. It was written by Lalanne, who commented in the editorial: 'It's said to be a risky business dealing with change and innovation. Fortunately, Sophie Marceau poses no threats for a cover, but the cigarette wedged in the corner of her apricot-coloured lips seriously divided the editorial staff and could prove to be a great deal more dangerous. Dangerous for the body, of course, but also dangerous for all those who are given to the pleasures of smoking a cigarette in public. We only have to look at the "outing" campaign launched in the United States by Smoke Free Movies against stars accused of promoting the consumption of tobacco. We have opted for the beauty of an image and for freedom. Aware, of course – and it can never be said too often – that smoking is bad for your health.' Lalanne is describing here *Vogue*'s current policy on its covers, which can be summed up in a few words: the impact of offbeat and surprising images and a plea for non-conformism and freedom. It is a policy to which the front cover of the May 2008 issue – featuring Julianne Moore in sexy and provocative mood – remains faithful.

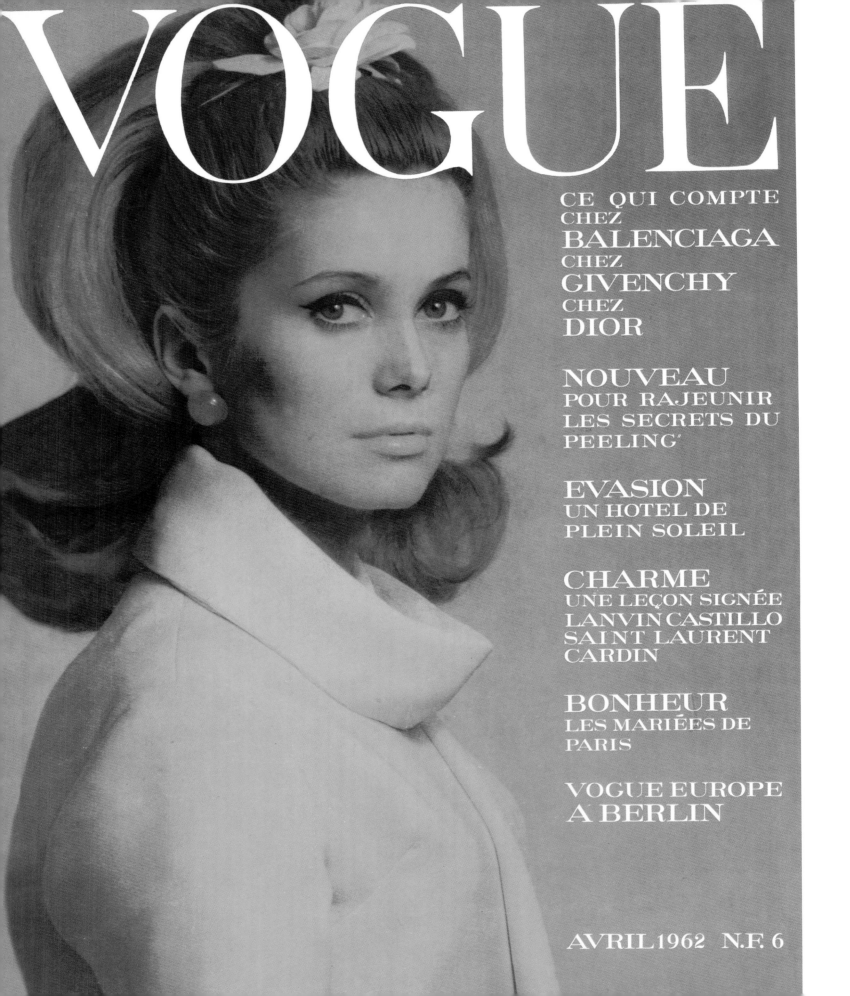

VOGUE

AVRIL 1962   N.F. 6

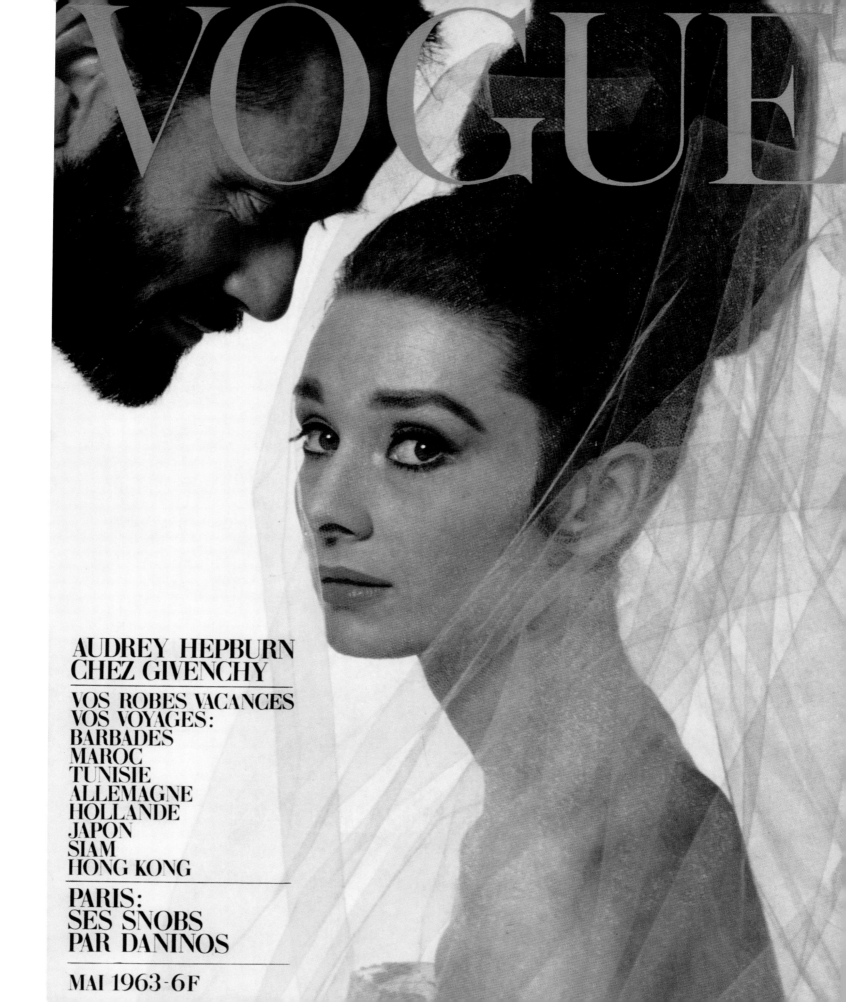

VOGUE

**AUDREY HEPBURN
CHEZ GIVENCHY**

VOS ROBES VACANCES
VOS VOYAGES:
BARBADES
MAROC
TUNISIE
ALLEMAGNE
HOLLANDE
JAPON
SIAM
HONG KONG

**PARIS:
SES SNOBS
PAR DANINOS**

MAI 1963 · 6F

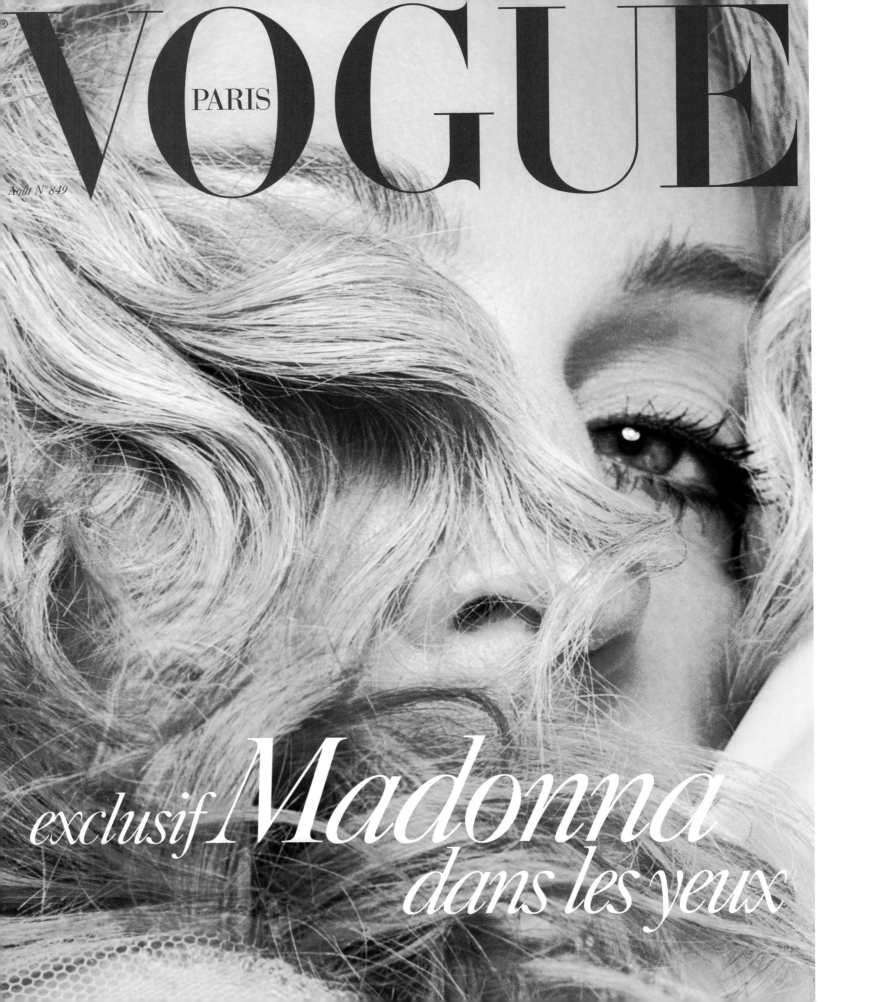

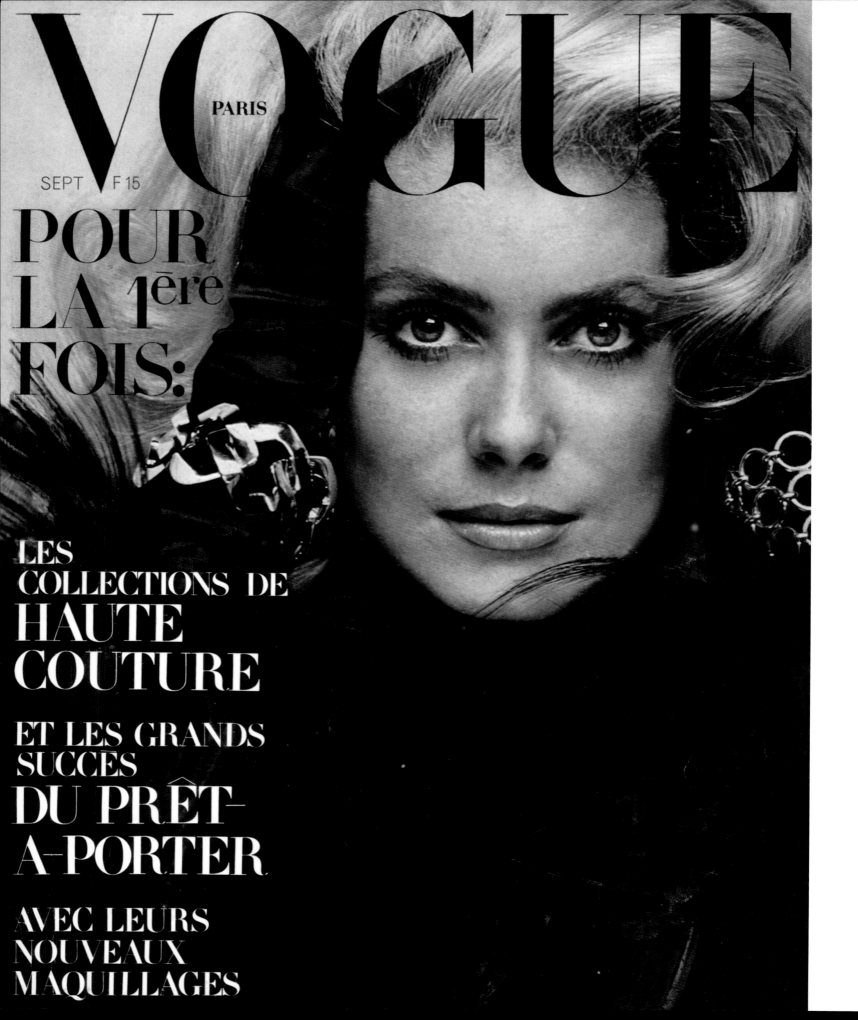

VOGUE

PARIS

SEPT F 15

POUR
LA 1ère
FOIS :

LES
COLLECTIONS DE
HAUTE
COUTURE

ET LES GRANDS
SUCCÈS
DU PRÊT-
A-PORTER

AVEC LEURS
NOUVEAUX
MAQUILLAGES

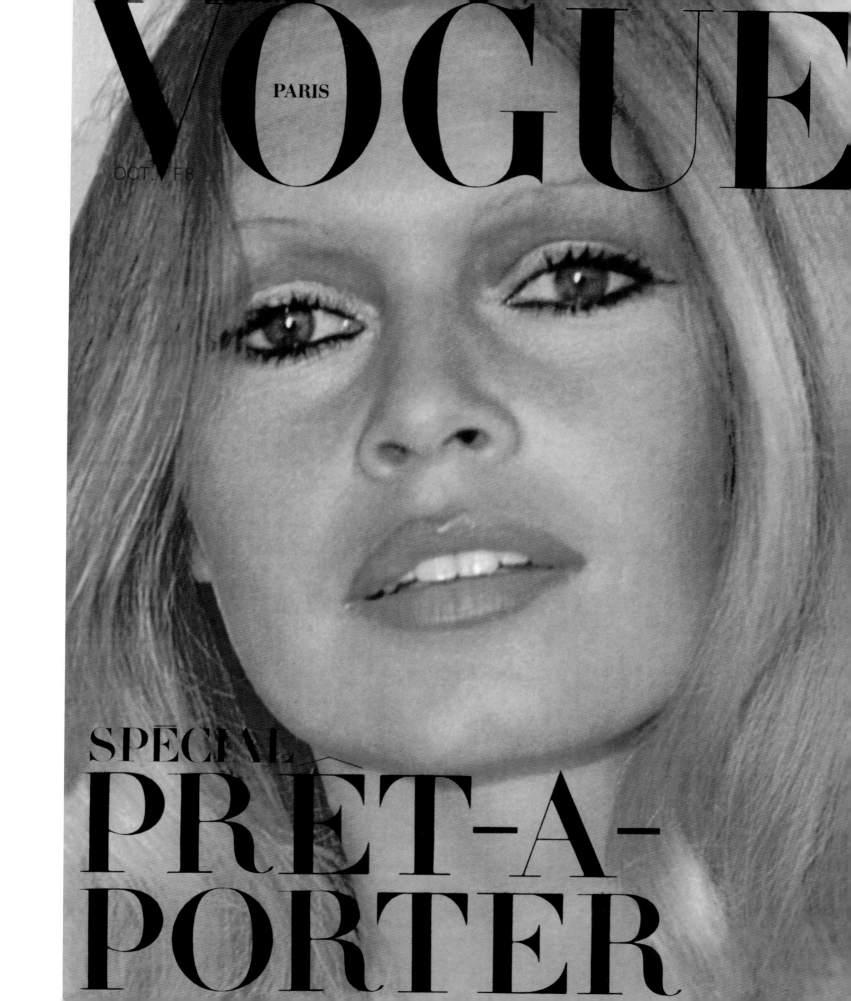

VOGUE

PARIS

OCT. VF 8

SPÉCIAL
PRÊT-A-
PORTER

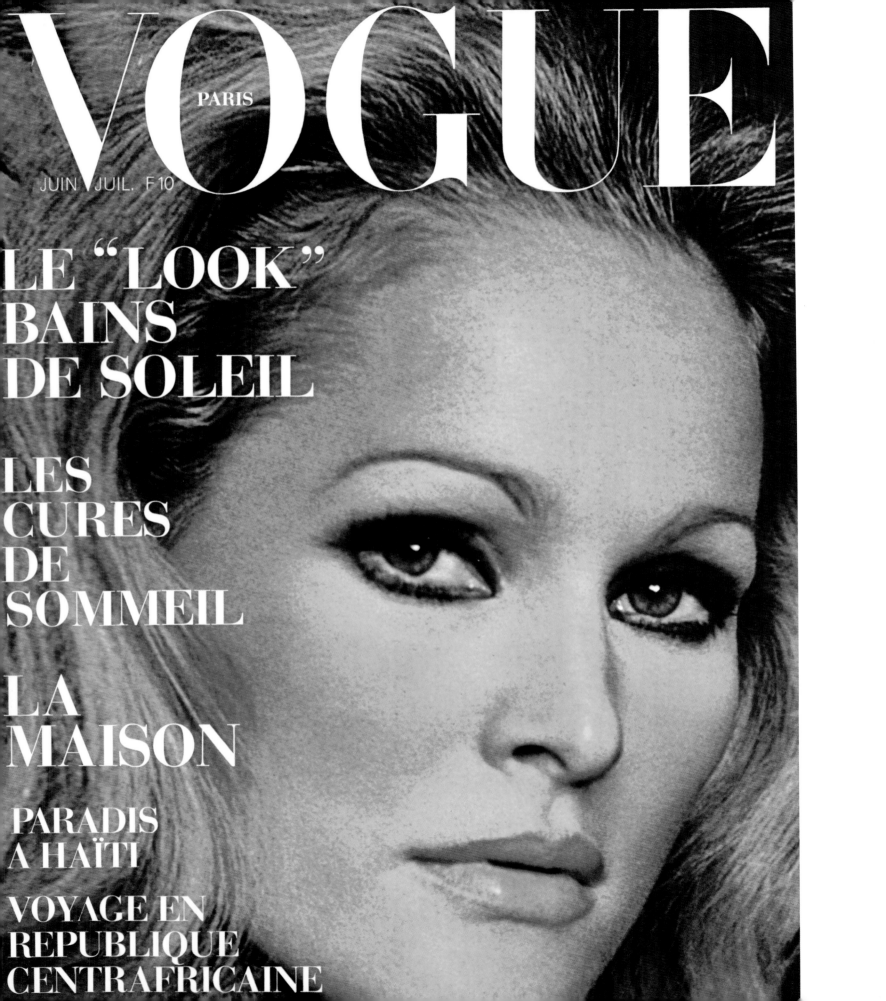

VOGUE PARIS

JUIN JUIL. F 10

LE "LOOK"
BAINS
DE SOLEIL

LES
CURES
DE
SOMMEIL

LA
MAISON

PARADIS
A HAÏTI

VOYAGE EN
REPUBLIQUE
CENTRAFRICAINE

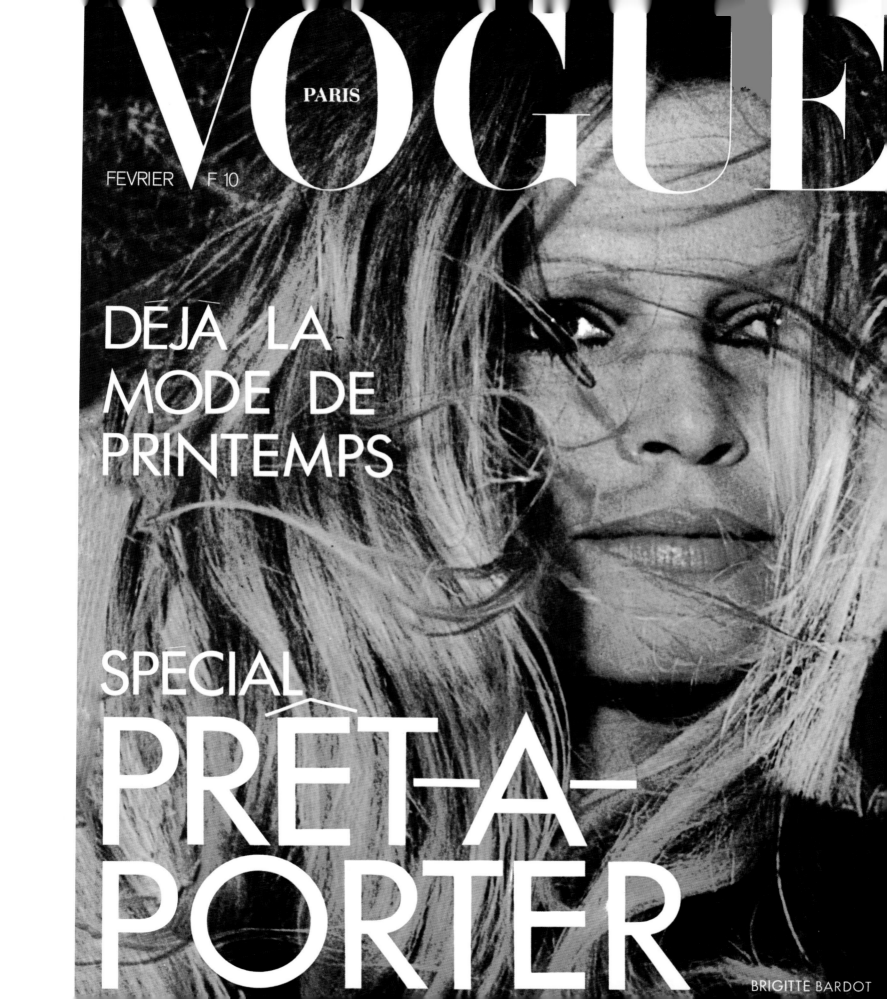

VOGUE
PARIS

FEVRIER   F 10

DÉJÀ LA MODE DE PRINTEMPS

SPÉCIAL
PRÊT-A-PORTER

BRIGITTE BARDOT

VOGUE

PARIS

SEPT. F 40

*LA
PRINCESSE
STEPHANIE
DE
MONACO*

PARIS
HAUTE COUTURE

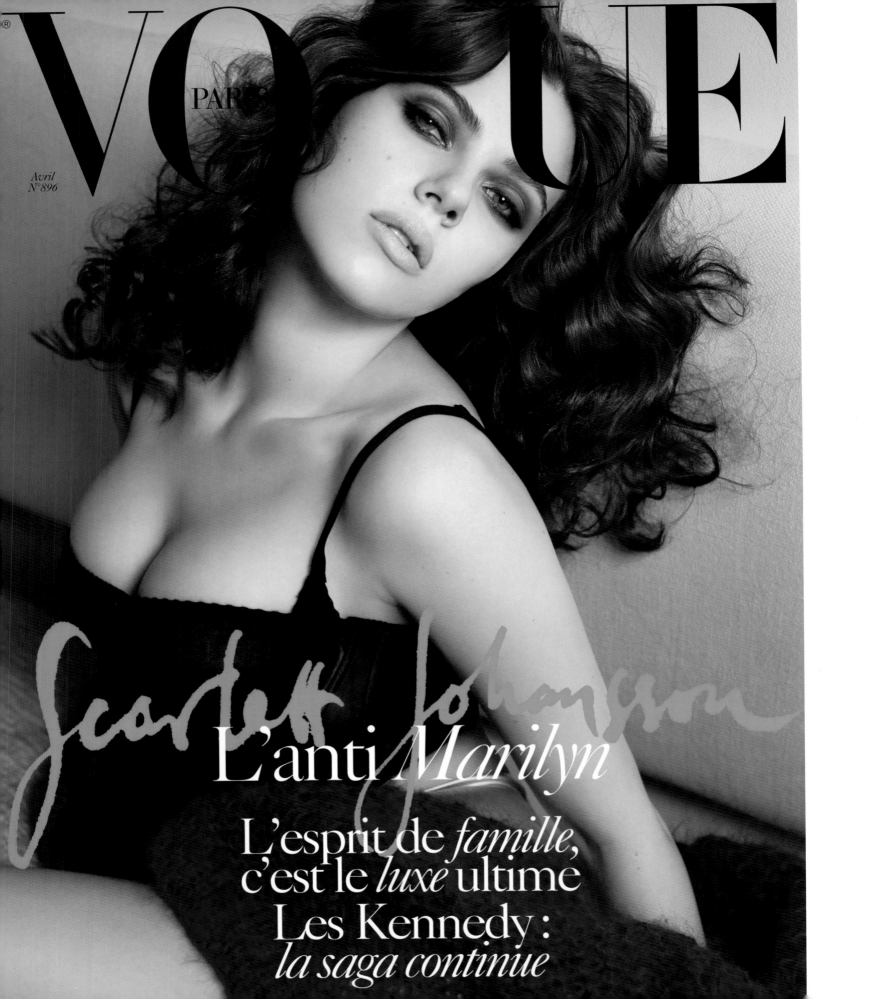

April 2009
Mario Sorrenti
Scarlett Johansson
Couturier Dolce & Gabbana

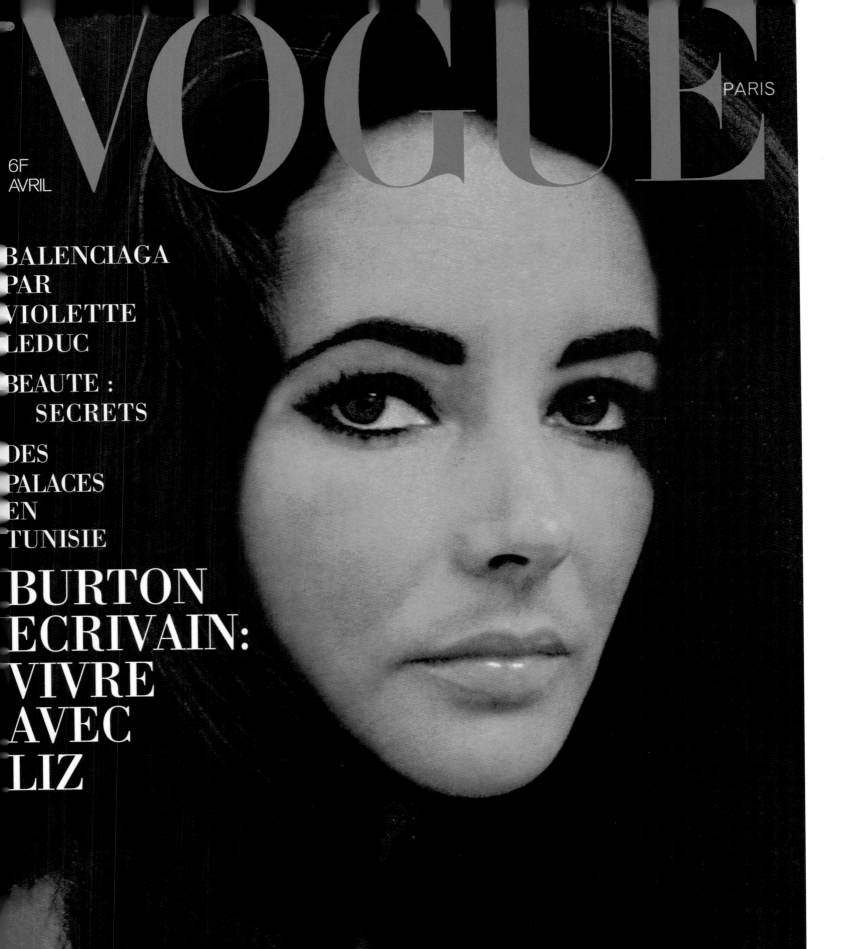

VOGUE
PARIS

6F
AVRIL

BALENCIAGA
PAR
VIOLETTE
LEDUC

BEAUTE :
  SECRETS

DES
PALACES
EN
TUNISIE

BURTON
ECRIVAIN:
VIVRE
AVEC
LIZ

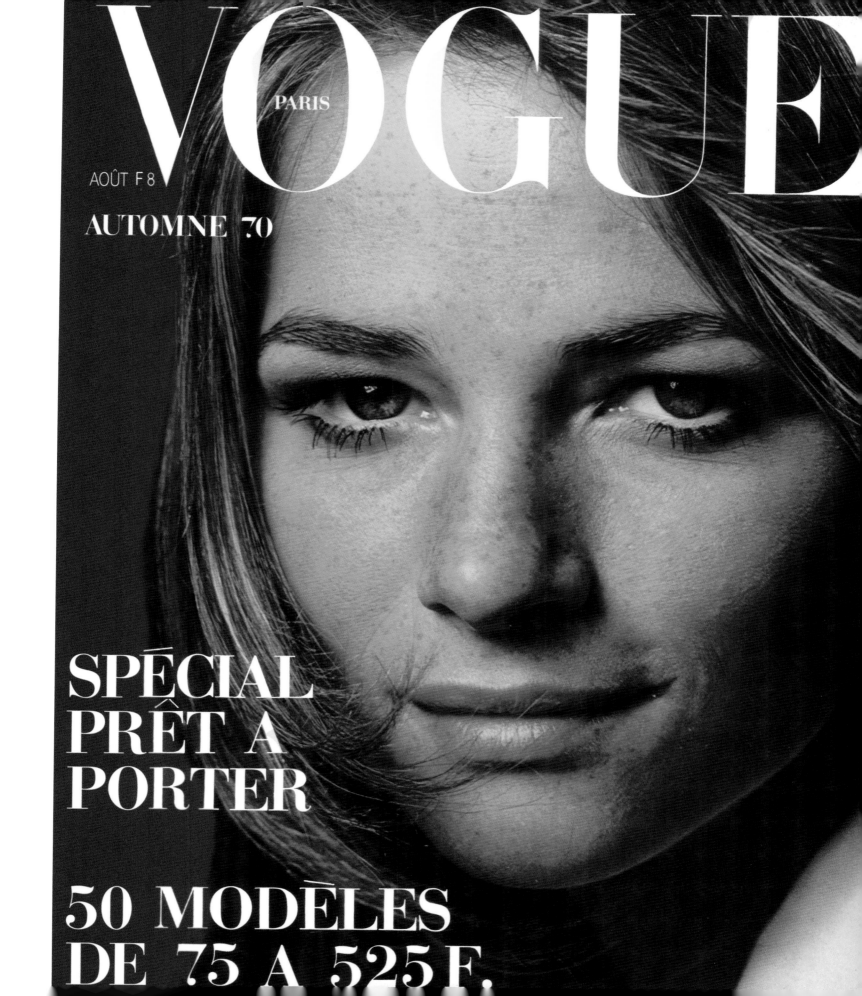

VOGUE

PARIS

AOÛT F 8

AUTOMNE 70

SPÉCIAL PRÊT À PORTER

50 MODÈLES DE 75 A 525 F.

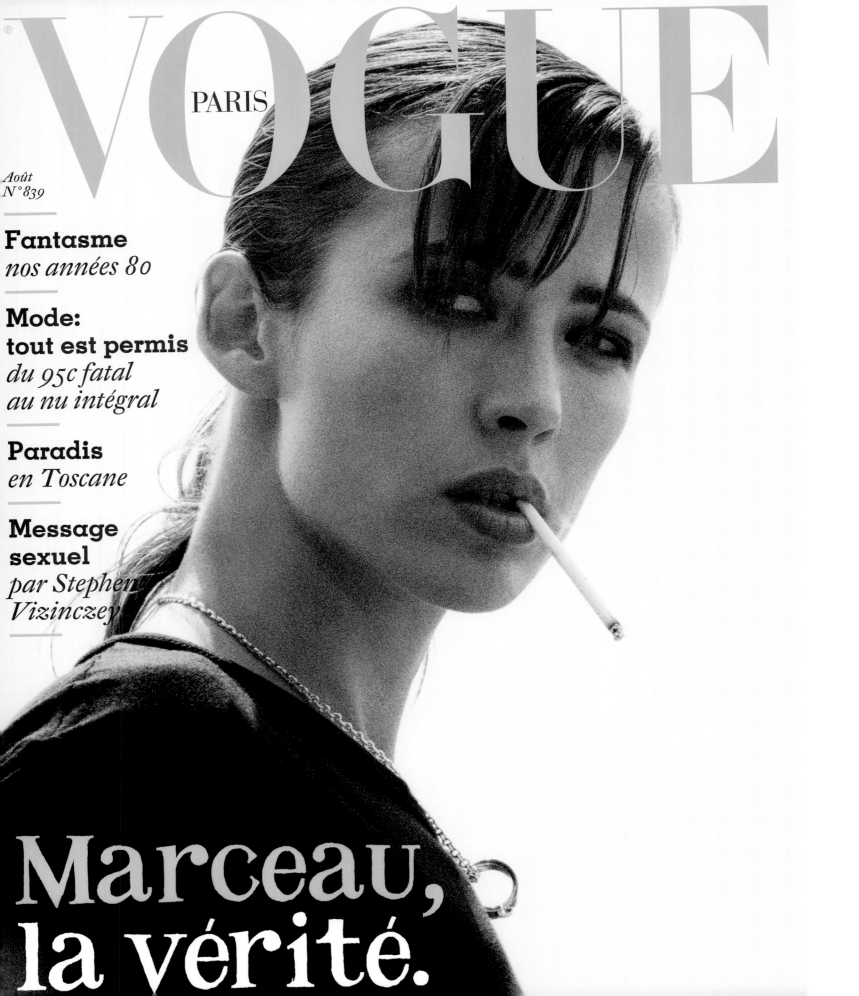

VOGUE PARIS

Août
N°839

Fantasme
nos années 80

Mode:
tout est permis
du 95c fatal
au nu intégral

Paradis
en Toscane

Message
sexuel
par Stephen
Vizinczey

Marceau,
la vérité.

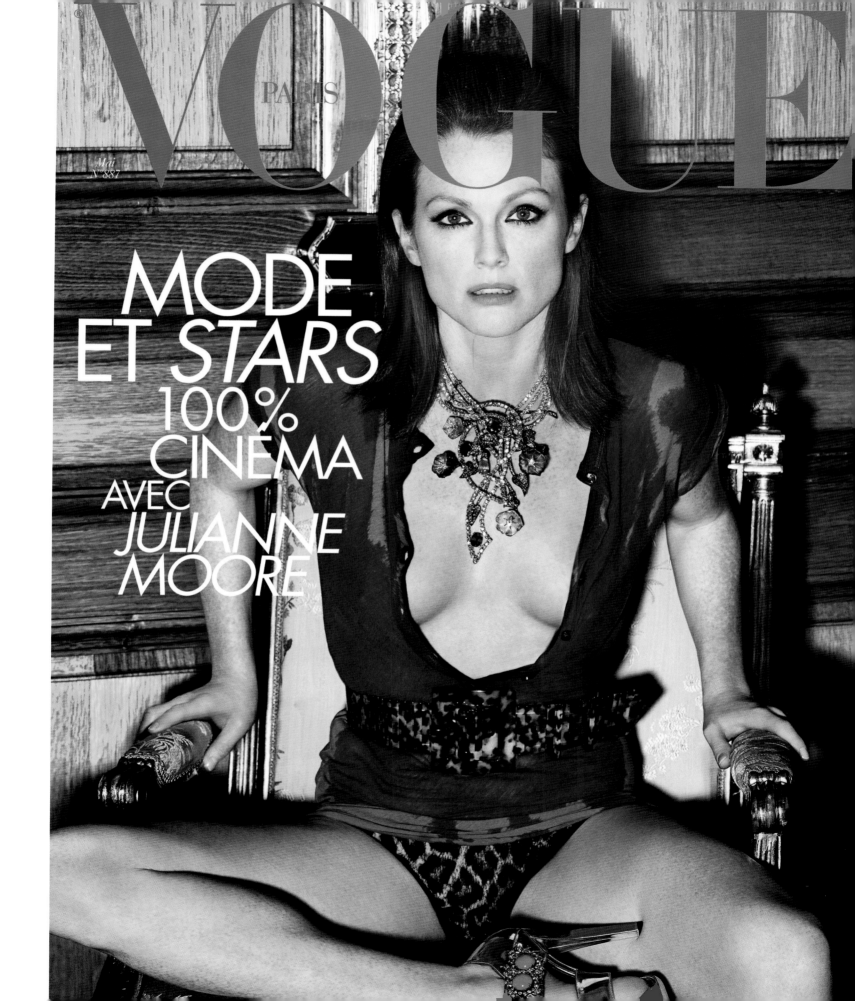

VOGUE
PARIS

Mai
N° 887

MODE
ET STARS
100%
CINÉMA
AVEC
JULIANNE
MOORE

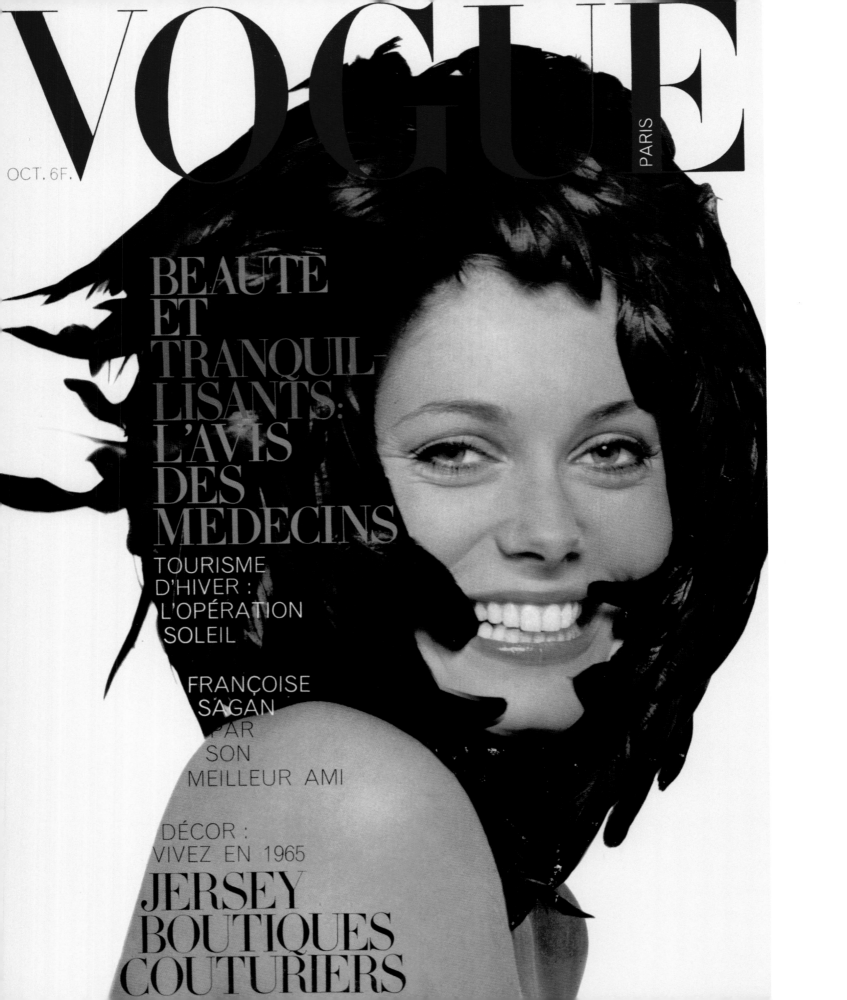

VOGUE

PARIS

OCT. 6F.

BEAUTÉ
ET
TRANQUIL-
LISANTS:
L'AVIS
DES
MÉDECINS

TOURISME
D'HIVER :
L'OPÉRATION
SOLEIL

FRANÇOISE
SAGAN
PAR
SON
MEILLEUR AMI

DÉCOR :
VIVEZ EN 1965

JERSEY
BOUTIQUES
COUTURIERS

The great outdoors

'Aside from gloves and stockings, the dress code for the country
is as detailed and as particular as that for the city.'
— *Vogue*, July–August 1951

The first issue of French *Vogue* in June 1920 bore on its cover an illustration by
Helen Dryden showing two women on a tennis court. The rackets and the net are
depicted, but the women's outfits are frankly unsuitable for physical exertion. The
tone was set: the aim of the new magazine was to reflect modern chic and the chic
side of modern life.

Contemporary chic, for the upper classes, meant decamping to their summer
residences in Le Touquet, Biarritz and Deauville and on the Riviera, centres of society
life where, one after another, the couturiers (privileged advertisers) began opening
boutiques. During the summer season, this was where it all happened – this was where
the fashionable and glamorous element of society spent their time – and, since this
was the society it served to mirror, *Vogue* naturally went there too.

The French tennis star, Suzanne Lenglen, then at the height of her career, was
the embodiment of all that was chic and modern, regarded as a national heroine by
the adoring elite with whom she also socialized. Thanks to Lenglen, who won every

international title (including Wimbledon and the French Championships) between 1919 and 1923, tennis became *the* celebrity sport. But Lenglen revolutionized the game not only through her play but also through her outfits, which included a daringly short pleated skirt (cut just below the knee), a pink hairband and a fur stole for her arrival on court.

Over and above their graphic qualities, this first cover by Helen Dryden and the cover designed by Georges W. Plank a little more than a year later in November 1921 are accurate illustrations of the interests and lifestyle of *Vogue*'s readers, for whom nature provided a familiar background for a fair amount of the year, but without greatly disrupting their urban habits. The scenery changed, but whether it was a question of chasing after a butterfly or wielding a tennis racket, the poses were rather indolent and appearances smart. Suzanne Lenglen was an icon, but as a sportswoman she was set apart upon a pedestal.

During the 1920s, the great outdoors such as it appeared on the front covers of *Vogue* was not so much the setting for a body exerting itself as for a holiday lifestyle. And in this respect substantial developments were to occur over the next decade. In fact, throughout its ninety-year existence, the covers of the magazine that take nature as their background – sea or mountains – tell us more than any others about the evolution of the *Vogue* woman, a woman from a wealthy milieu whose way of life, aspirations and relationship with beauty and well-being were constantly evolving and harmonizing with the trends and movements of successive eras.

During the 1930s, she was to be found, for example, sailing a yacht or riding on the back of a camel – in other words, active, moving, determined, the engaging centre of holiday life. In ten years, she had come a long way, a woman of the world who also intended henceforth to play her part in the world. This was very much the course taken by Chanel, who made it fashionable to have a suntan instead of keeping one's skin pale at all costs as a sign of allegiance to the leisured classes. As skin began to be exposed, clothes became more energetic and exercise fashionable. Nevertheless, with paid holidays just around the corner, and sport quietly but surely becoming more democratic, the elite inevitably sought new ways to set themselves apart. If leisure-time activities were to be available to virtually anyone, the elite would aspire to adventure instead – to travel and more thrilling activities that simultaneously offered an escape from an age over which the shadow of the 1929 economic crisis still hung. And when in November 1938 a hunting party featured on the front cover of *Vogue*, the objective remained the same: no question of the mundane, the everyday, the round of popular pastimes; if being beautiful meant you had to move about, and toning up meant developing muscles, then let it be done in the most glamorous and romantic way possible, like in a Hollywood film. Being chic was not a question of sitting back and resting.

The 1950s by contrast were years of physical relaxation, of sensuality, of the smile, as associated with models such as Grace Kelly, Brigitte Bardot, Sophia Loren and Marilyn Monroe. After the endless privations of wartime, the mood was now resolutely materialistic and pleasure-oriented. People enjoyed what they could, and laughed about the rest: 'The importance of futile things' ran the headline to a January 1945 editorial by Claude Blanchard. Whether she was looking aristocratic at the races, sporty on a mountain top, or relaxed and natural by the sea, the *Vogue* woman as depicted on its covers gained humour and realism and shed some of her haughty aloofness. The adventures were over; now the focus was on holidays, on relaxing and enjoying one's freedom – a freedom that was all the more precious since the rest of one's time was devoted to work. *Vogue* woman was now an active woman, for whom elegance was combined with a sense of physical well-being and an element of practicality. Since daily life brought its own constraints, there was no question of imposing too many more on herself when it came to relaxing and having fun – and the poses in the photographs are more relaxed too. The 1950s were a turning point for the magazine. While it was now centred more around Paris, as we saw in the last chapter, it had no intention of cutting itself off from its provincial readership: the top fashion labels sold reproduction rights and other licences to couturiers operating in the big cities throughout France, and it was important to keep them happy. So the magazine regularly included lengthy articles relating to other areas of France, offering a mixture of fashion and culture that was reflected in covers with a reportage feel, or anchored at any rate in 'real life' situations. Here we find, for example, a series of articles entitled '*Vogue*'s views on the development of tourist fashion'.

From the 1960s onwards, the outdoors element of the covers produced a more eclectic landscape, a picture album illustrating the habits and lifestyle of the typical *Vogue* woman certainly, but also more general developments in beauty and fashion towards an increasingly 'bare' look. The idea of escape came to be embodied by sea and sand, that highly evocative environment that reflected the evolution of a lifestyle from both a physical and a mental perspective. It was more than an aesthetic. It was a landscape rich in symbols – freedom, health, purity, lightness, sunlight. And it was a perfect canvas on which to display, successively, the 1960s ideal of natural beauty, the expansiveness of the 1970s, the 1980s focus on performance, and the fixation on health and well-being that was the hallmark of the 1990s. In every instance, *Vogue*'s covers reflected the spirit of the magazine, a magazine that championed active, independent, international women – who were not afraid to jump in the water.

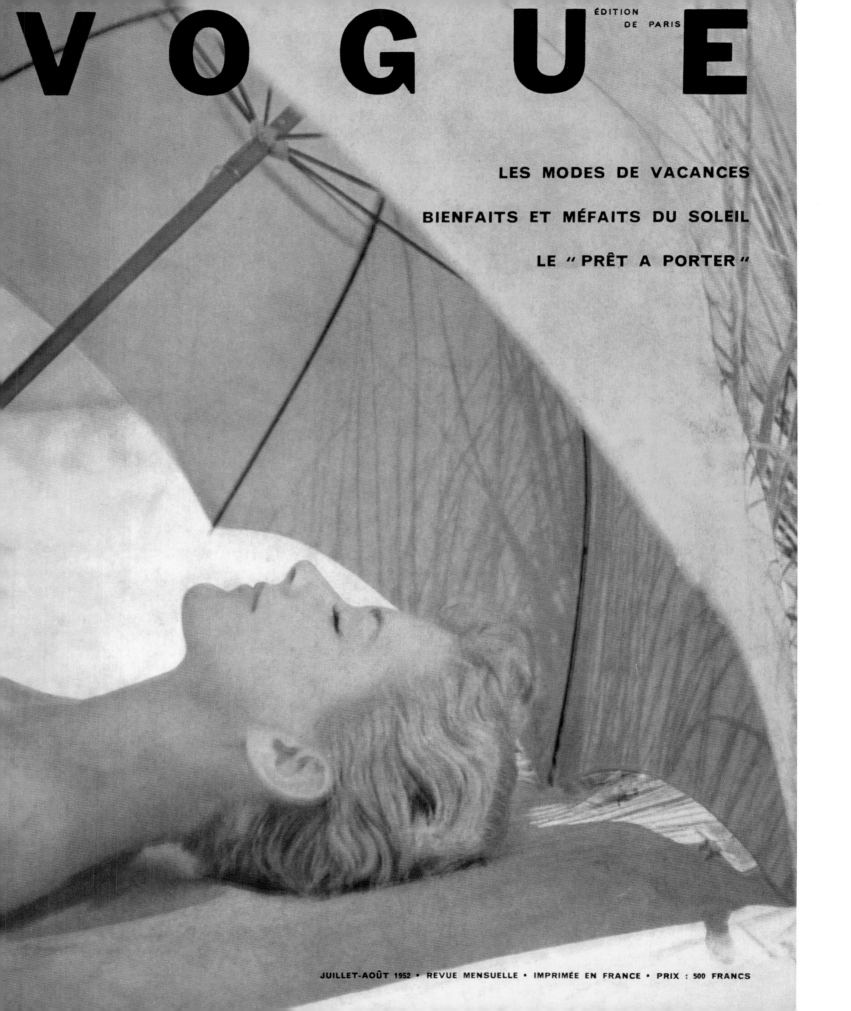

VOGUE

ÉDITION DE PARIS

LES MODES DE VACANCES

BIENFAITS ET MÉFAITS DU SOLEIL

LE « PRÊT A PORTER »

JUILLET-AOÛT 1952 • REVUE MENSUELLE • IMPRIMÉE EN FRANCE • PRIX : 500 FRANCS

July–August 1952
Irving Penn

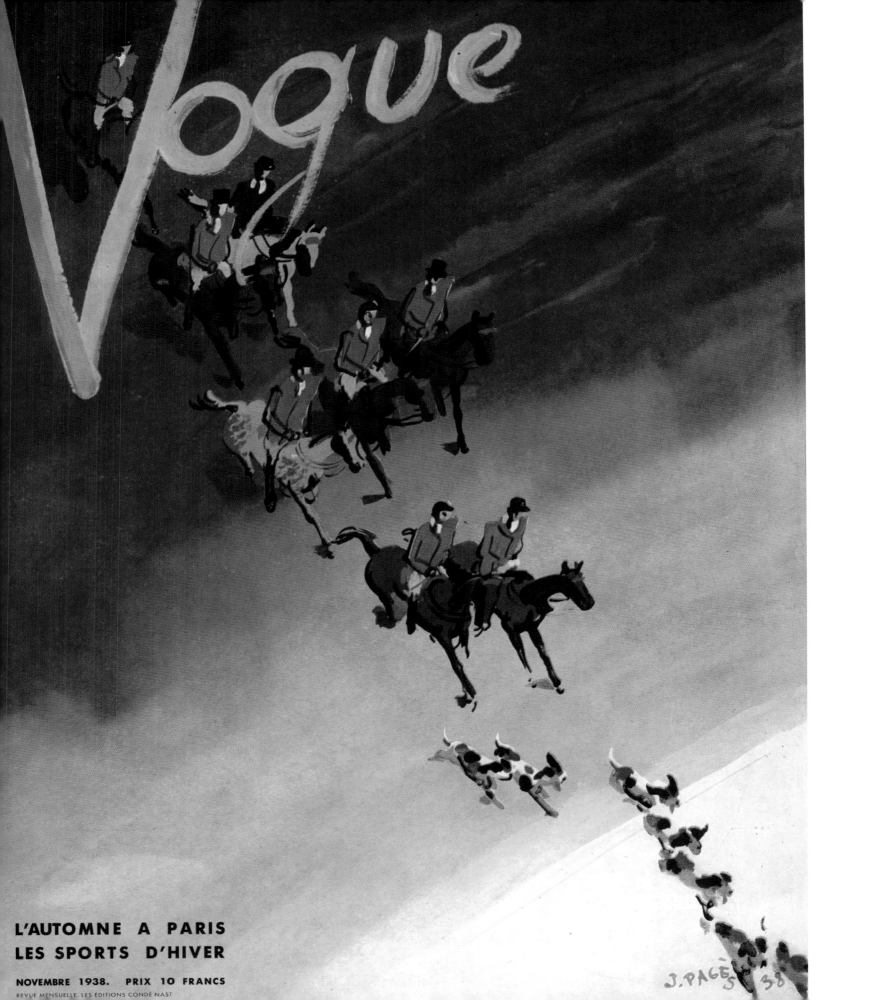

Vogue

L'AUTOMNE A PARIS
LES SPORTS D'HIVER

NOVEMBRE 1938. PRIX 10 FRANCS

REVUE MENSUELLE. LES ÉDITIONS CONDÉ NAST

J.PAGÈS 38

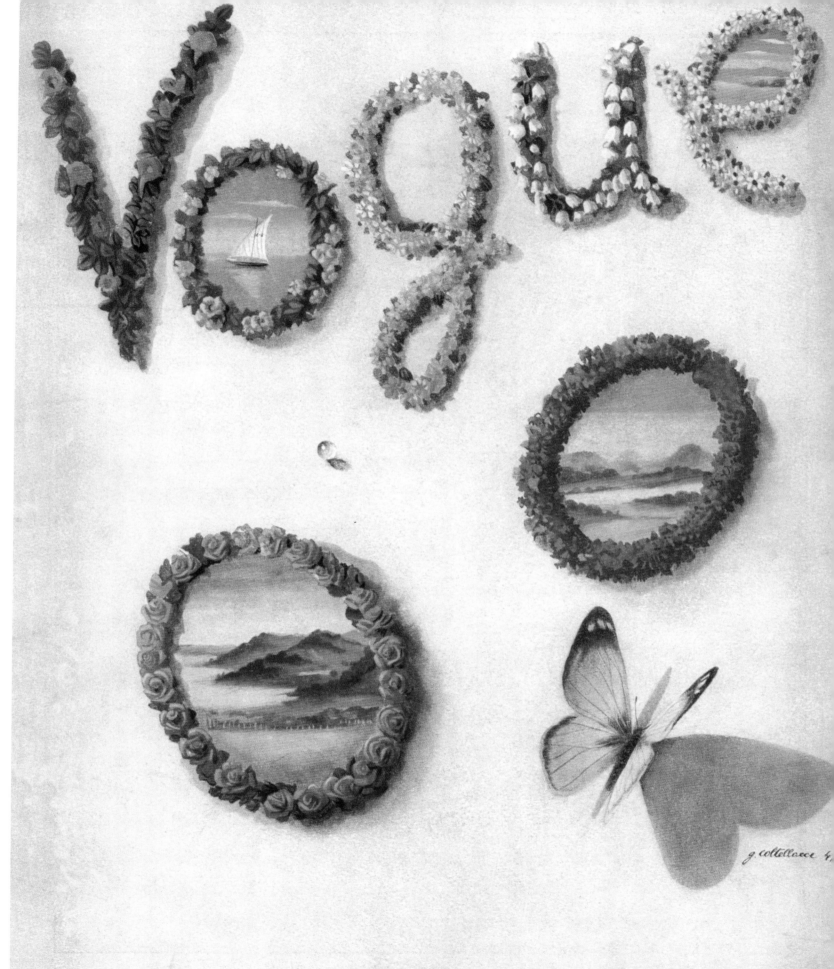

JUILLET-AOÛT 1947   PUBLICATION BIMESTRIELLE   PRIX : 180 FRANCS
IMPRIMÉE EN FRANCE

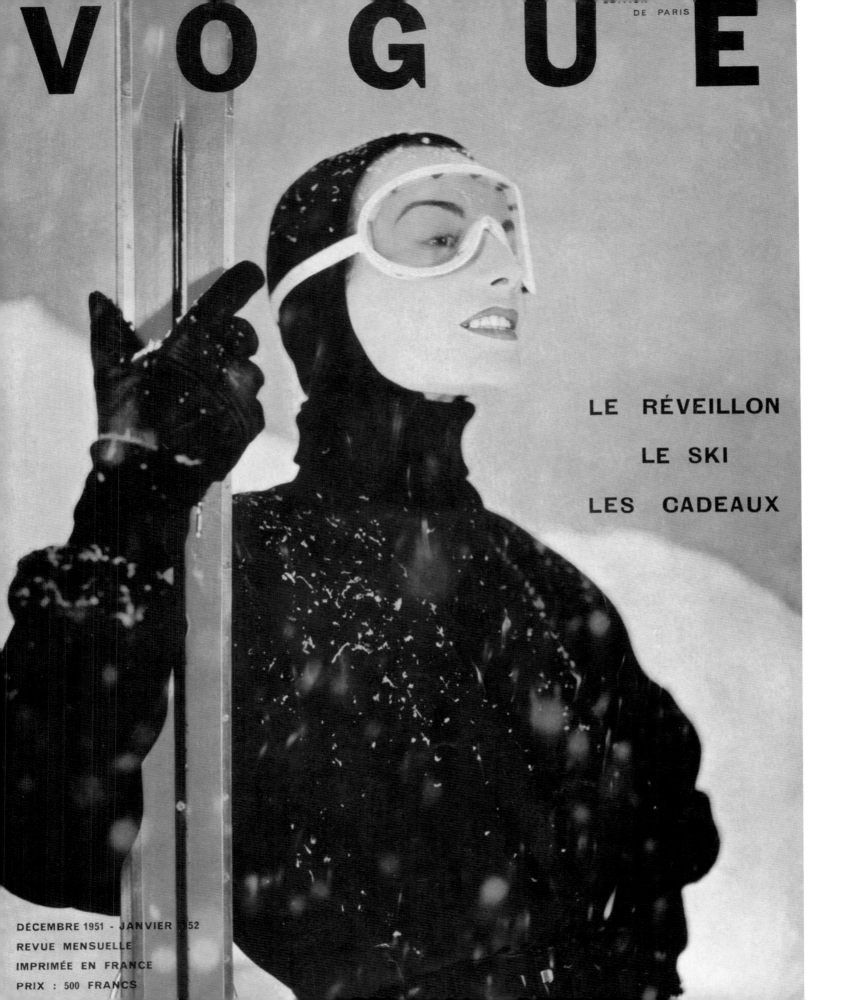

VOGUE

EDITION DE PARIS

LE RÉVEILLON

LE SKI

LES CADEAUX

DÉCEMBRE 1951 - JANVIER 1952

REVUE MENSUELLE

IMPRIMÉE EN FRANCE

PRIX : 500 FRANCS

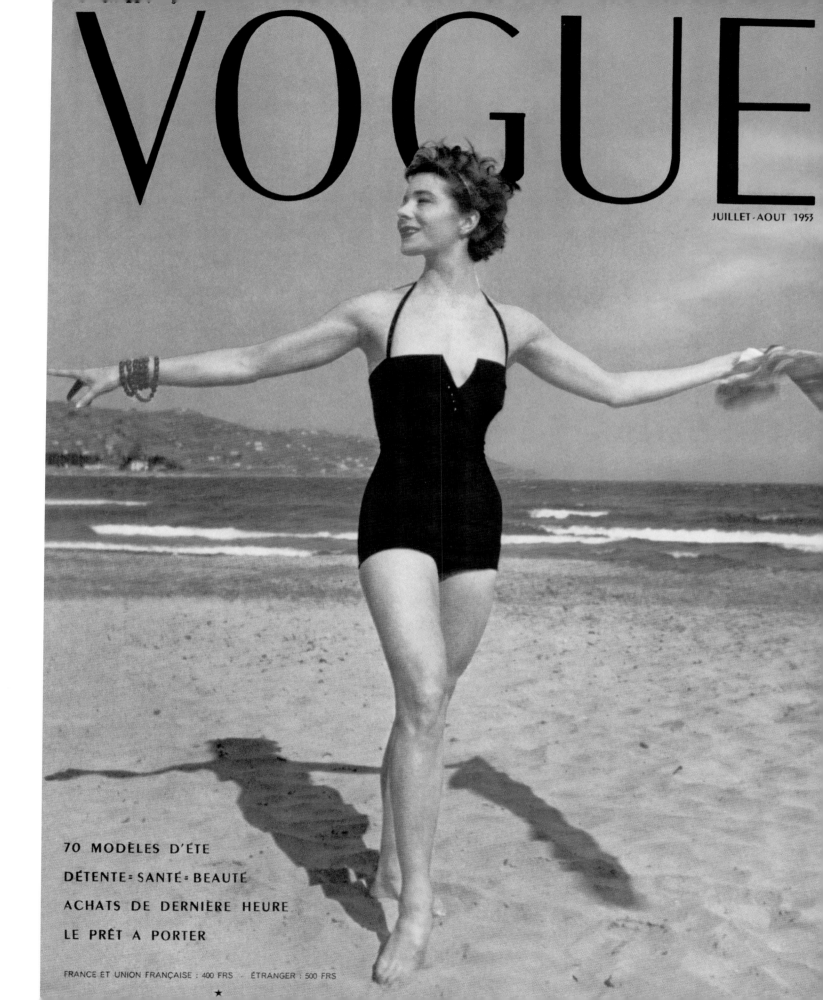

VOGUE

JUILLET-AOUT 1953

70 MODÈLES D'ÉTÉ

DÉTENTE = SANTÉ = BEAUTÉ

ACHATS DE DERNIÈRE HEURE

LE PRÊT A PORTER

FRANCE ET UNION FRANÇAISE : 400 FRS · ÉTRANGER : 500 FRS

★

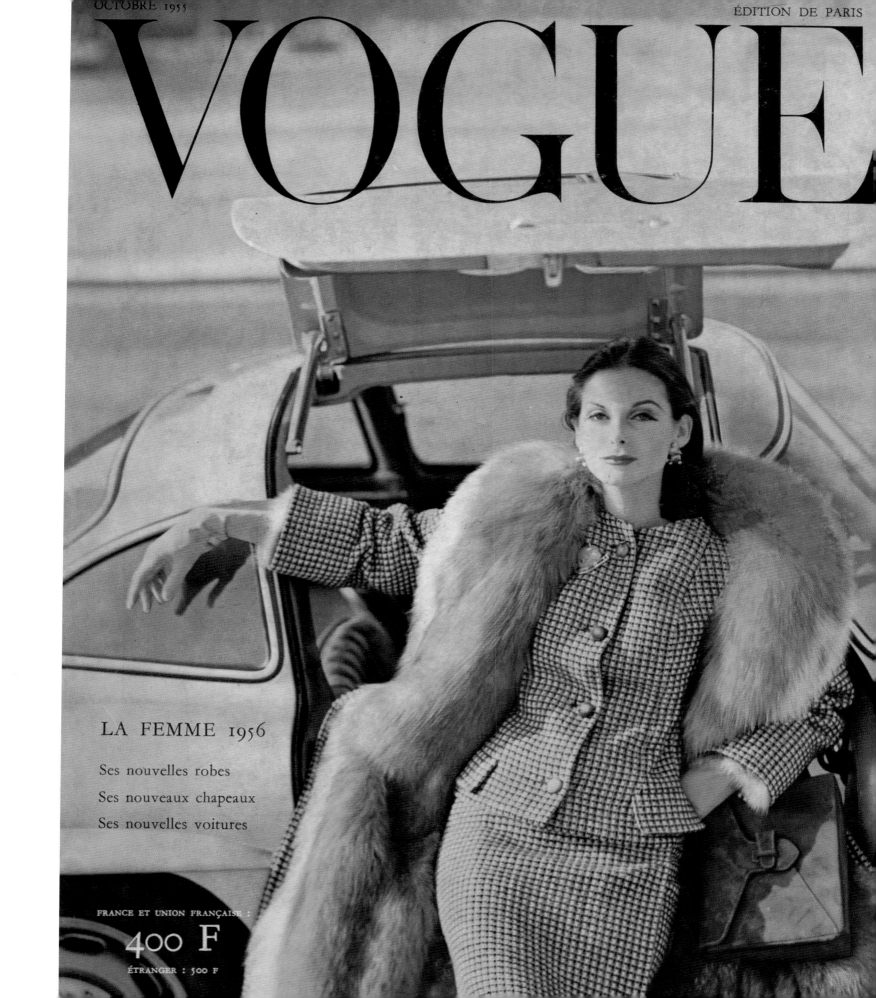

OCTOBRE 1955

ÉDITION DE PARIS

VOGUE

LA FEMME 1956

Ses nouvelles robes

Ses nouveaux chapeaux

Ses nouvelles voitures

FRANCE ET UNION FRANÇAISE :

400 F

ÉTRANGER : 500 F

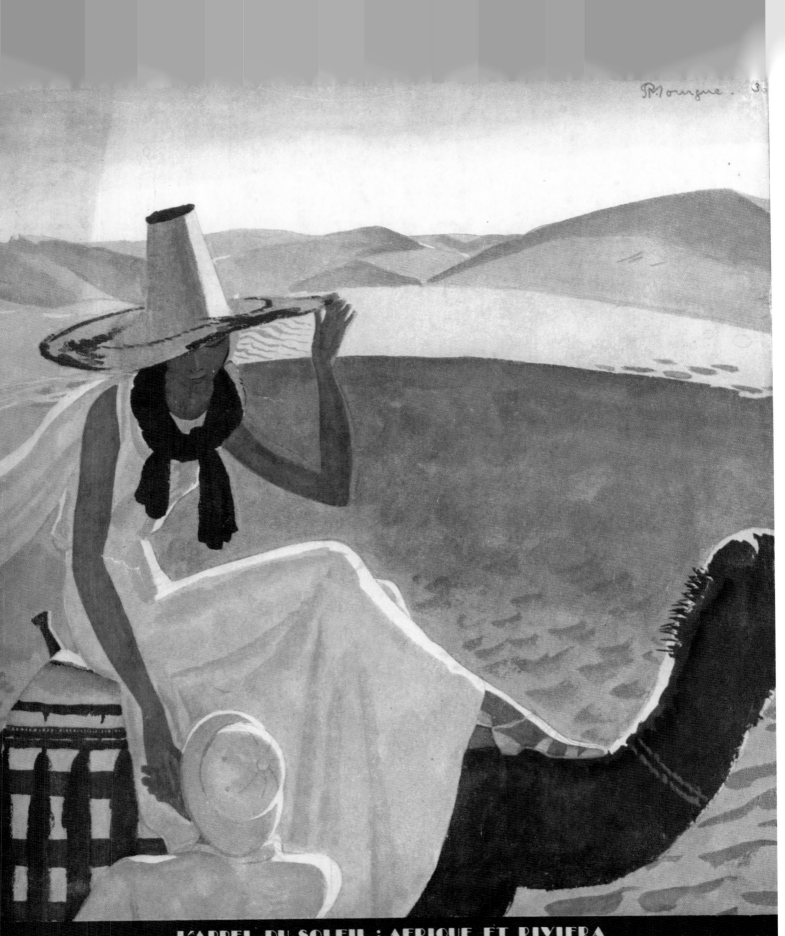

PRIX: 6 FRANCS   L'APPEL DU SOLEIL : AFRIQUE ET RIVIERA   JANVIER 1931
CONFIRMATION DE LA MODE · DE LA LINGERIE

VOGUE

JUIN 1950. REVUE MENSUELLE IMPRIMÉE EN FRANCE. PRIX : 400 FRS

LES
COLLECTIONS
DE
PLEIN ÉTÉ

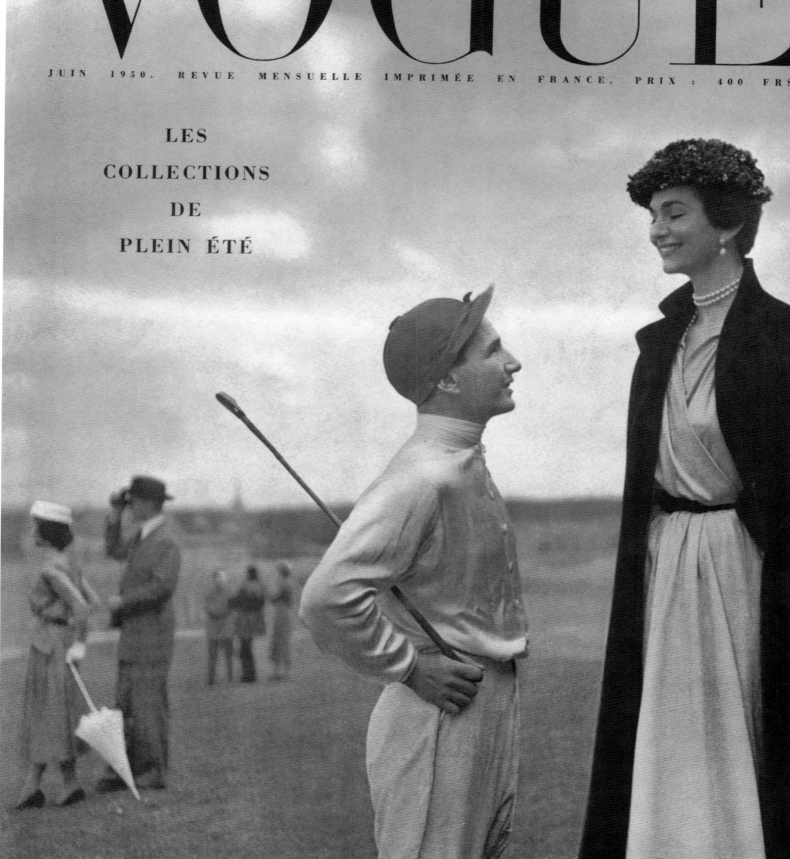

PREVIOUS PAGES
January 1931
Pierre Mourgue

June 1950
Robert Randall

OPPOSITE
June 1964
Helmut Newton

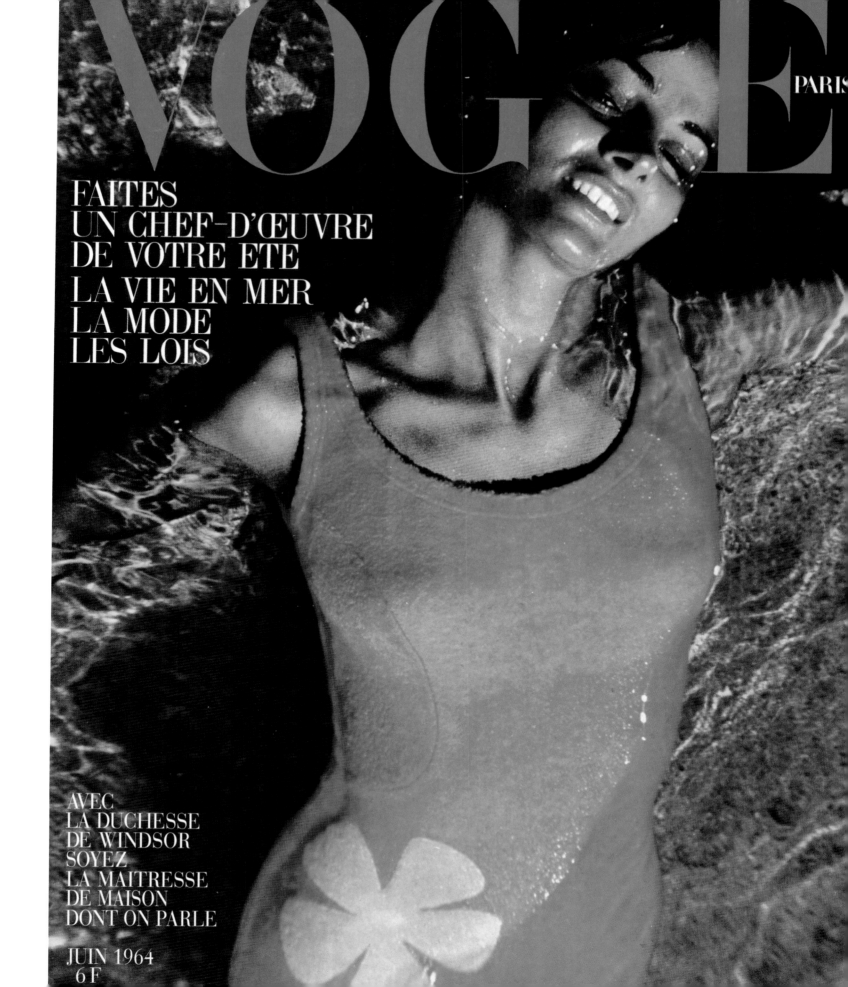

VOGUE

PARIS

FAITES
UN CHEF-D'ŒUVRE
DE VOTRE ÉTÉ
LA VIE EN MER
LA MODE
LES LOIS

AVEC
LA DUCHESSE
DE WINDSOR
SOYEZ
LA MAÎTRESSE
DE MAISON
DONT ON PARLE

JUIN 1964
6 F

On with the show!

'Elegance is refusal.'
— Diana Vreeland

'Art is tremendously adaptable. It is as much at ease in *Vogue*
as on the walls of a museum or gallery.'
— Edward Steichen

Vogue is eccentric. *Vogue* is funny, non-conformist, different. *Vogue* is provocative and avant-garde; it breaks with convention. '*Vogue* does not really fit with feminine types of things in the traditional sense of the word. It has no wish to remain on the highway of "right-mindedness" or "good taste". Its covers sometimes look like an aesthetic coup d'état, as if they were gambling primarily on the image that they will leave behind,' comments Olivier Lalanne, Assistant Editor of *Vogue* since 2006. What that means in practice is that some of these covers deliberately break the established rules for an 'effective' cover – legibility, pleasing headlines, attractive colours, direct eye contact, appealing fashions… A recent example, the November 2008 issue, shows a barely recognizable Vanessa Paradis, looking utterly different from the way we know her, in close-up with the smallest headline. In choosing between an image in which the star is clearly recognizable – an argument in favour of increased sales – and taking a chance on an outstanding photo – signed Mert Alas & Marcus Piggott – likely to be of lasting interest, *Vogue* has opted for aesthetic value. The willingness to take this risk – the risk, in other words, of losing sales in a context governed by the dynamic of profitability – has long been the magazine's particular hallmark, although it does not always and necessarily yield to the temptation of the powerful image to the detriment of the more commercial one.

The break with convention is all the more striking for not being routine. *Vogue* continues to be a magazine that focuses on luxury, fashion and contemporary art, and it is precisely as such that it is able legitimately, and on occasion, to break the rules by flaunting a daring and unexpected cover. In fact, this risk-taking also belongs to the worlds of luxury, fashion and contemporary art, universes where transgression is a right, even an obligation. Over the years, this element of risk has continued to take a variety of forms. It may be embodied in the almost clownish energy of a Tom Keogh or the appealingly child-like vision of an André François, who in the immediate post-war years fostered a playful and faux-naïve style of drawing – the expression of a rediscovered freedom but also of the uncertainties and privations experienced by the fashion world at that time – when expectations inclined in fact towards something more glamorous. The risk was also embodied, in the 1960s, in the graphic power of unusual layouts and of photographs signed by Richard Avedon and Guy Bourdin which reconnected with the idea of seeing the funny side of things, making self-mockery the expression of feminine liberation. It was also embodied in the wax dummy signed by Helmut Newton (March 1978), which took the place of a real flesh-and-blood model, producing a powerful and disconcerting physical metamorphosis that prefigured the covers of the 1980s; and, more recently, in the figure of the transvestite, whose presence on the cover of the November 2007 issue pushed the genre to its very limits; and, more generally, in the urge to flout 'good form' as understood by the middle classes.

The most committed *Vogue* covers, radical presentations that are willing to flaunt their difference and to take the criticism that goes with it – these are the covers that live on (even if, on the whole, greater moderation is required on the cover than on the pages inside the magazine). They are the covers that endure in people's memories, as they do in this book, going beyond their role as 'advertising' and acquiring a value that is altogether less transitory. Edward Steichen – chief photographer for Condé Nast in the 1920s – was right, it seems, when he maintained that commercial pressure would prove an amazingly productive force.

September 1965
David Bailey
Couturier
Yves Saint Laurent
'Mondrian Dress'

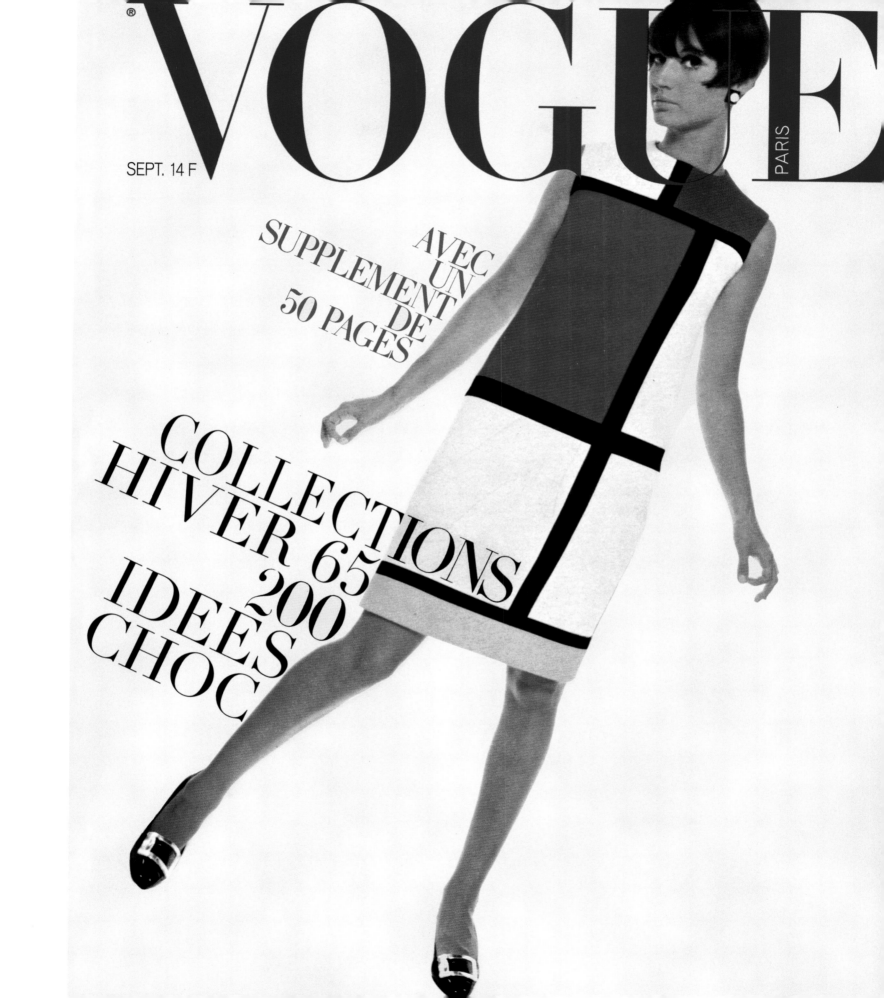

VOGUE

PARIS

SEPT. 14 F

AVEC UN SUPPLEMENT DE 50 PAGES

COLLECTIONS
HIVER 65
200
IDEES
CHOC

Vogue

Prix : 300 frs

Septembre 1948. Publication mensuelle. Imprimée en France

André François

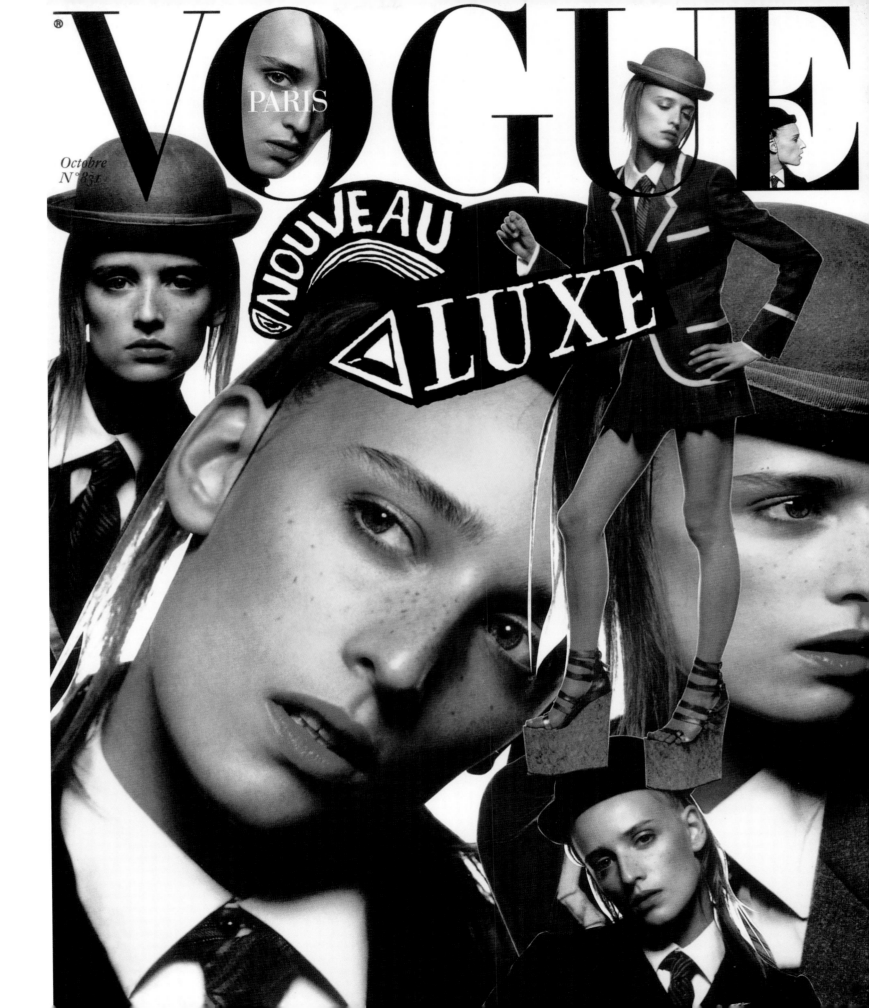

VOGUE

PARIS

Octobre
N° 831

NOUVEAU
VOGUE
LUXE

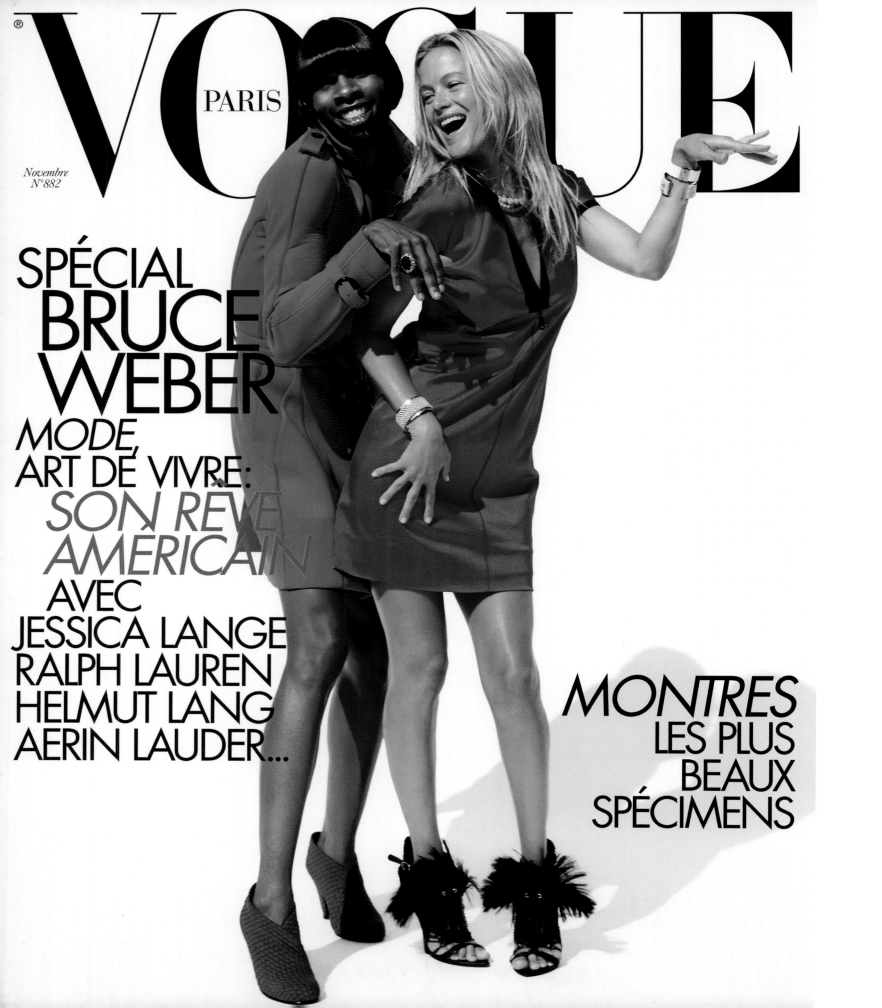

VOGUE

PARIS

Novembre
N°882

SPÉCIAL
BRUCE
WEBER
MODE,
ART DE VIVRE:
SON RÊVE
AMERICAIN
AVEC
JESSICA LANGE
RALPH LAUREN
HELMUT LANG
AERIN LAUDER...

MONTRES
LES PLUS
BEAUX
SPÉCIMENS

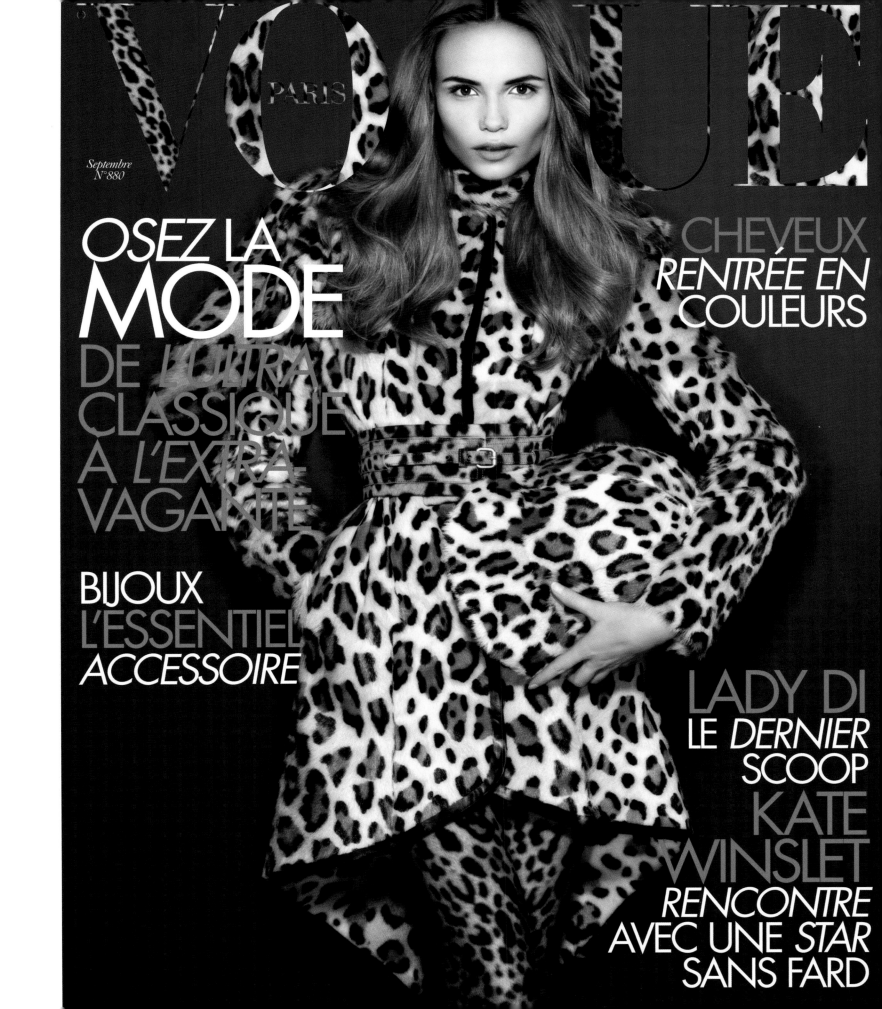

VOGUE

PARIS

Septembre
N°880

OSEZ LA
MODE

DE *L'ULTRA*
CLASSIQUE
À *L'EXTRA-*
VAGANTE

BIJOUX
L'ESSENTIEL
ACCESSOIRE

CHEVEUX
RENTRÉE EN
COULEURS

LADY DI
LE *DERNIER*
SCOOP

KATE
WINSLET
RENCONTRE
AVEC UNE *STAR*
SANS FARD

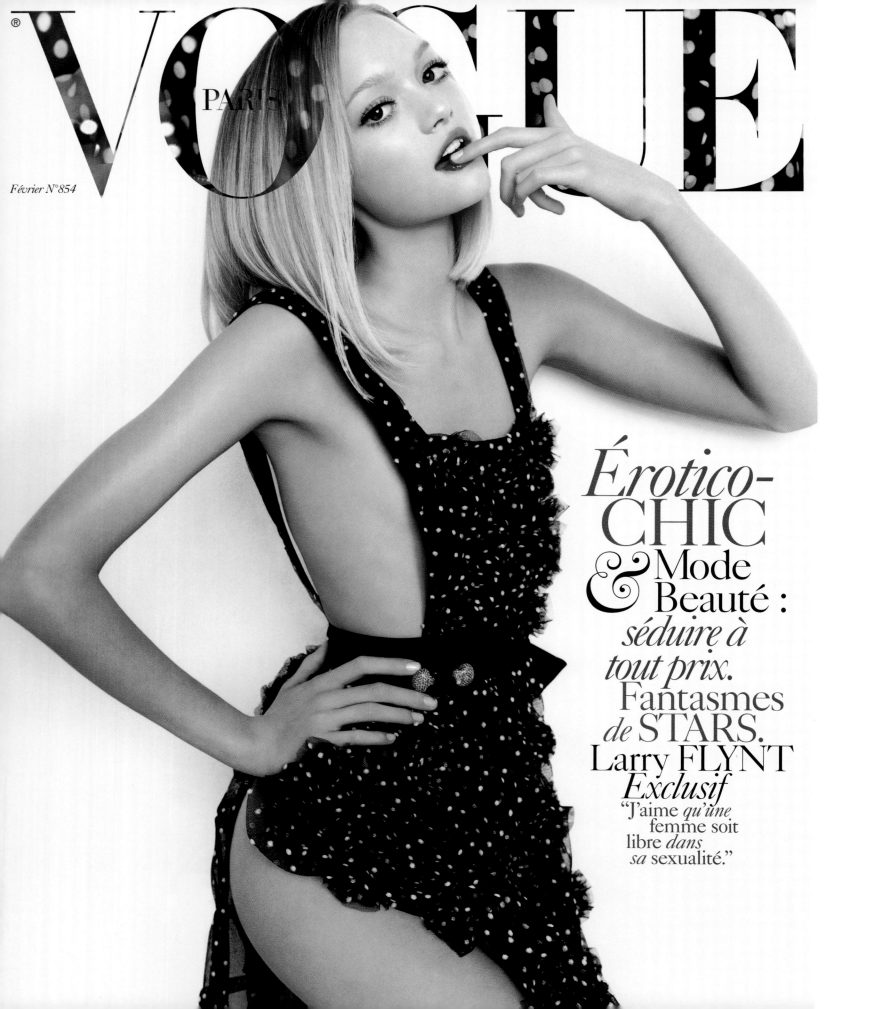

VOGUE

PARIS

Février N°854

Érotico-
CHIC
& Mode
Beauté :
*séduire à
tout prix.*
Fantasmes
de STARS.
Larry FLYNT
Exclusif
"J'aime *qu'une*
femme soit
libre *dans*
sa sexualité."

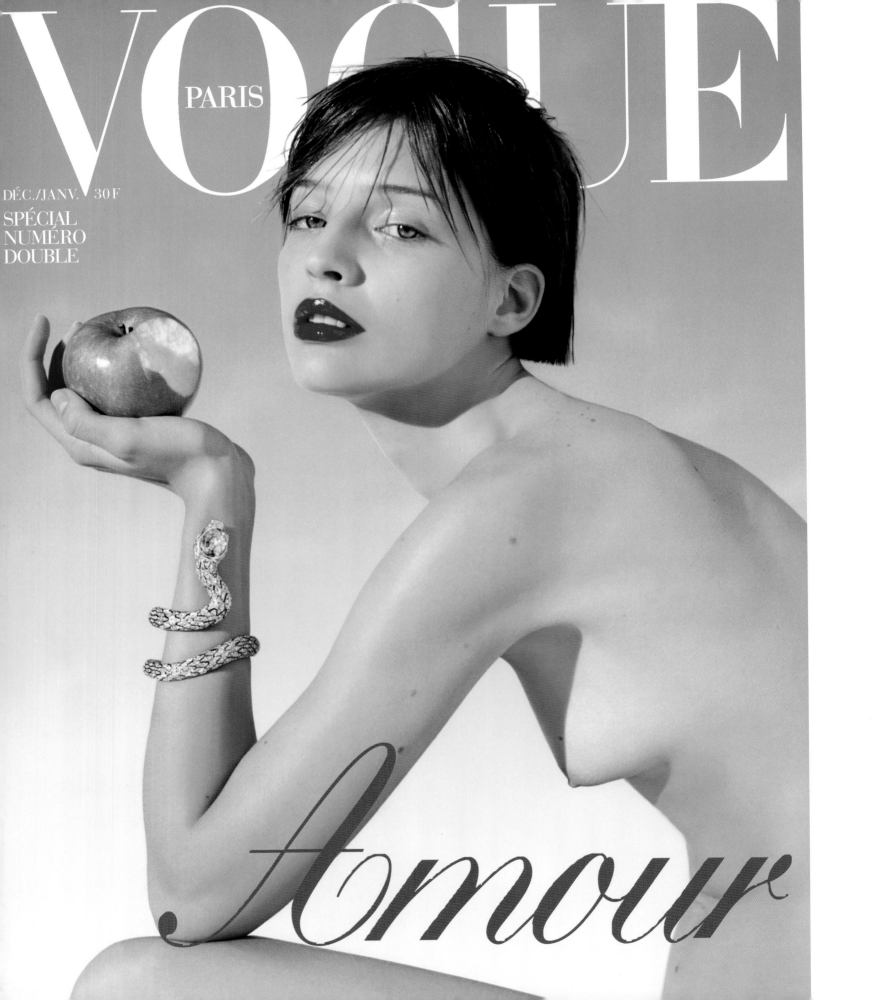

VOGUE PARIS

DÉC./JANV. 30 F

SPÉCIAL
NUMÉRO
DOUBLE

Amour

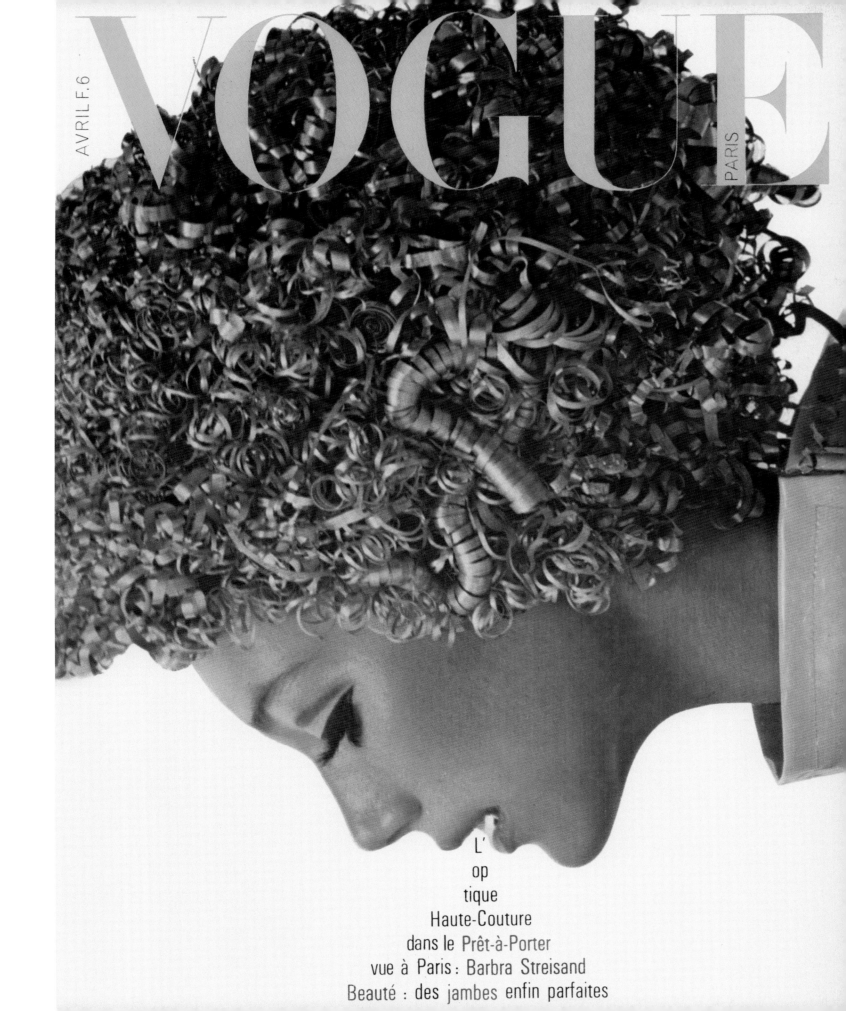

VOGUE

AVRIL F.6

PARIS

L'
op
tique
Haute-Couture
dans le Prêt-à-Porter
vue à Paris: Barbra Streisand
Beauté : des jambes enfin parfaites

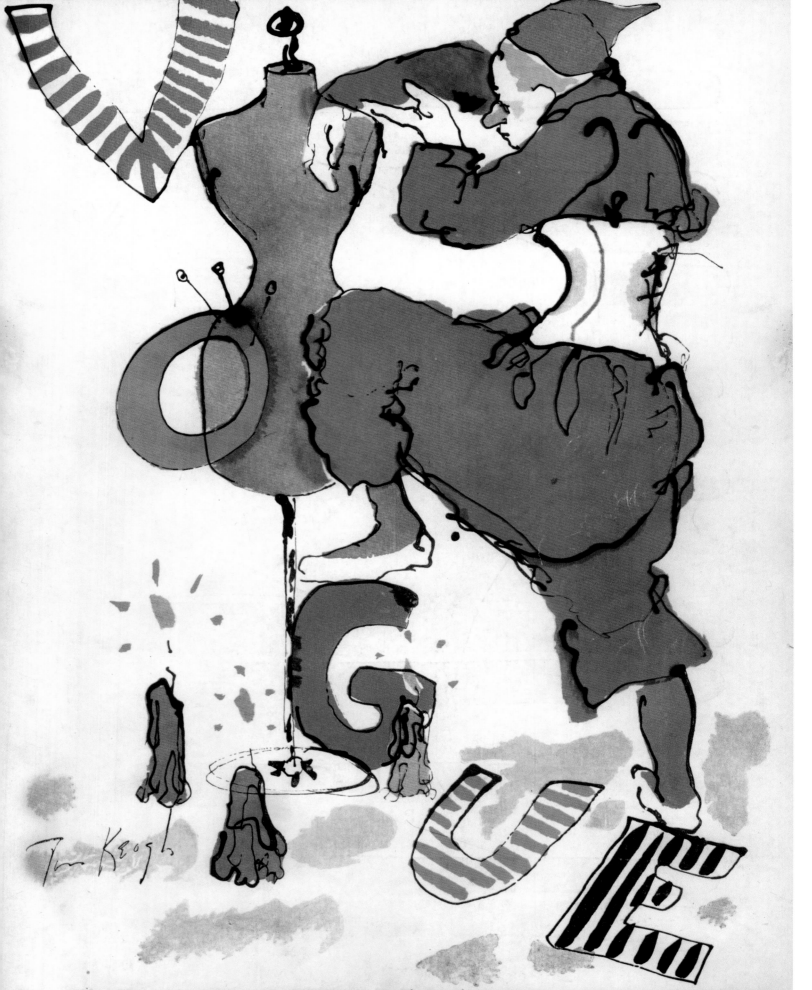

PRIX: 250 FRANCS — PUBLICATION BIMESTRIELLE — NUMÉRO SPÉCIAL DE DÉCEMBRE — IMPRIMÉE EN FRANCE

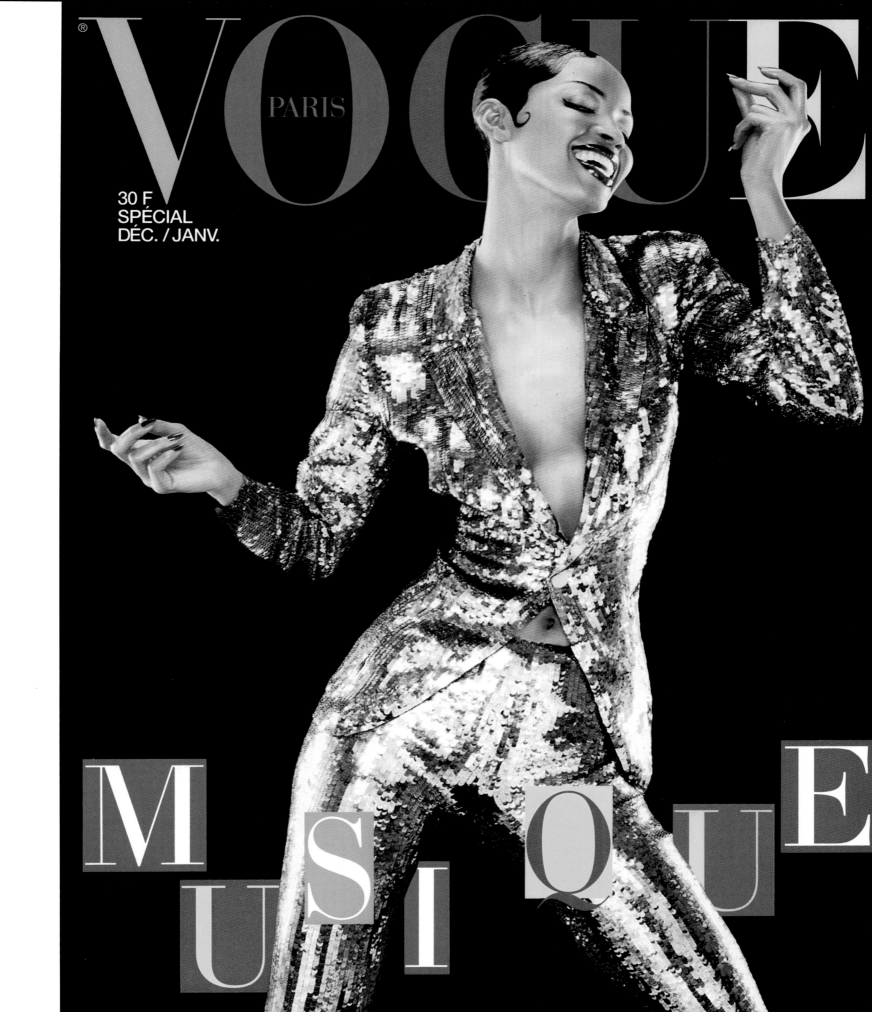

VOGUE

PARIS

30 F
SPÉCIAL
DÉC. / JANV.

MUSIQUE

PREVIOUS PAGES
December 1999
Jean-Baptiste Mondino
Model Linda Nyvltova
Jeweler Cartier

April 1966
Richard Avedon

December 1947
Tom Keogh

December 1996
Jean-Baptiste Mondino
Model Georgianna Robertson
Couturier Jean Paul Gaultier

OPPOSITE
November 2003
Inez van Lamsweerde
& Vinoodh Matadin
Model Diana Dondoe
Jeweler Van Cleef & Arpels
Couturier Gucci

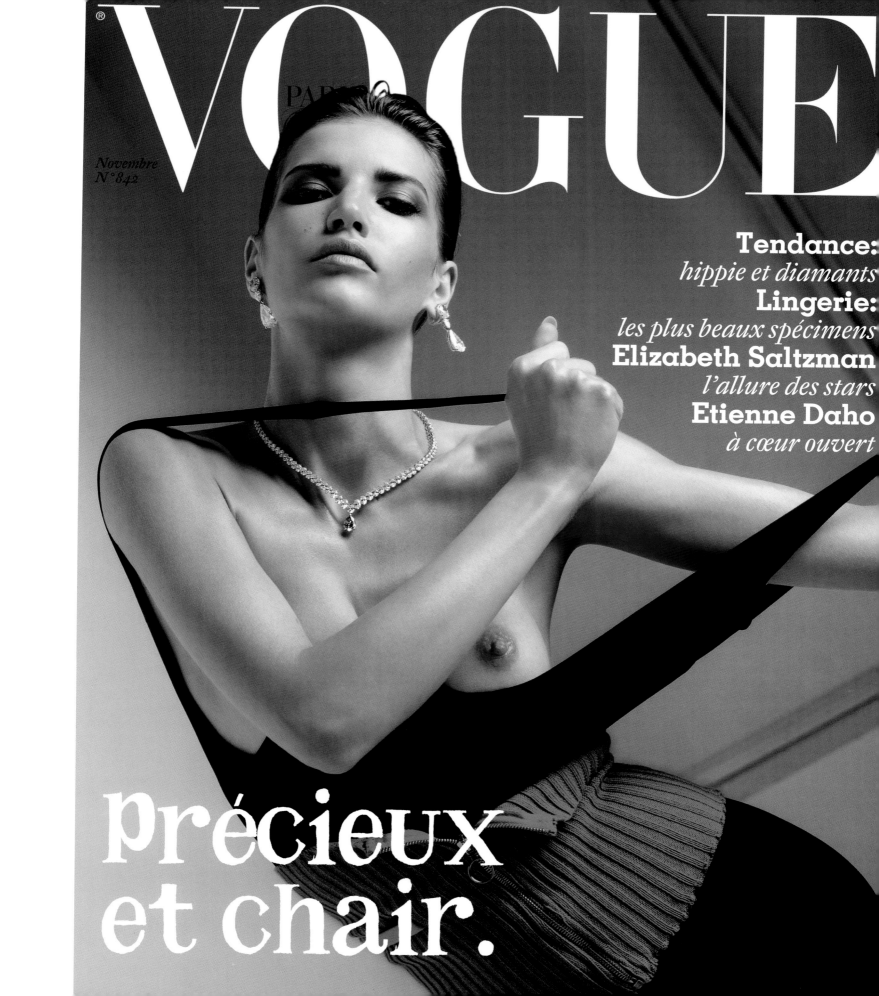

VOGUE

PARIS

Novembre
N° 842

Tendance:
hippie et diamants
Lingerie:
les plus beaux spécimens
Elizabeth Saltzman
l'allure des stars
Etienne Daho
à cœur ouvert

précieux
et chair.

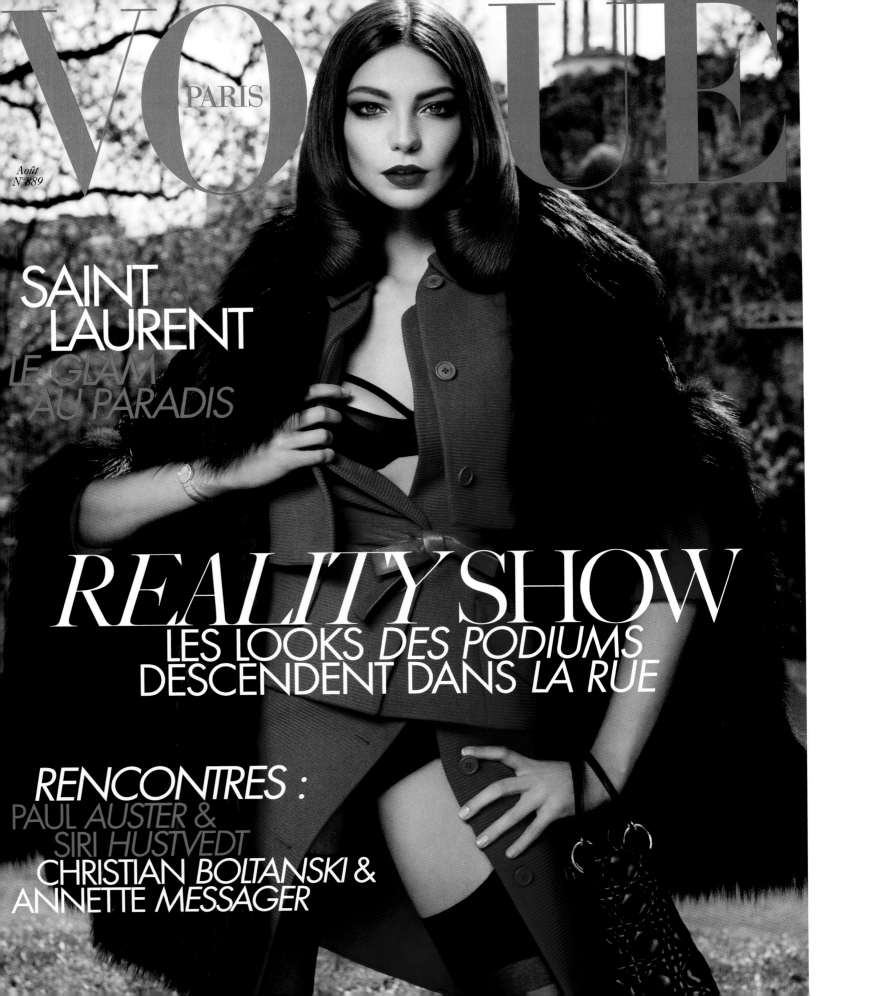

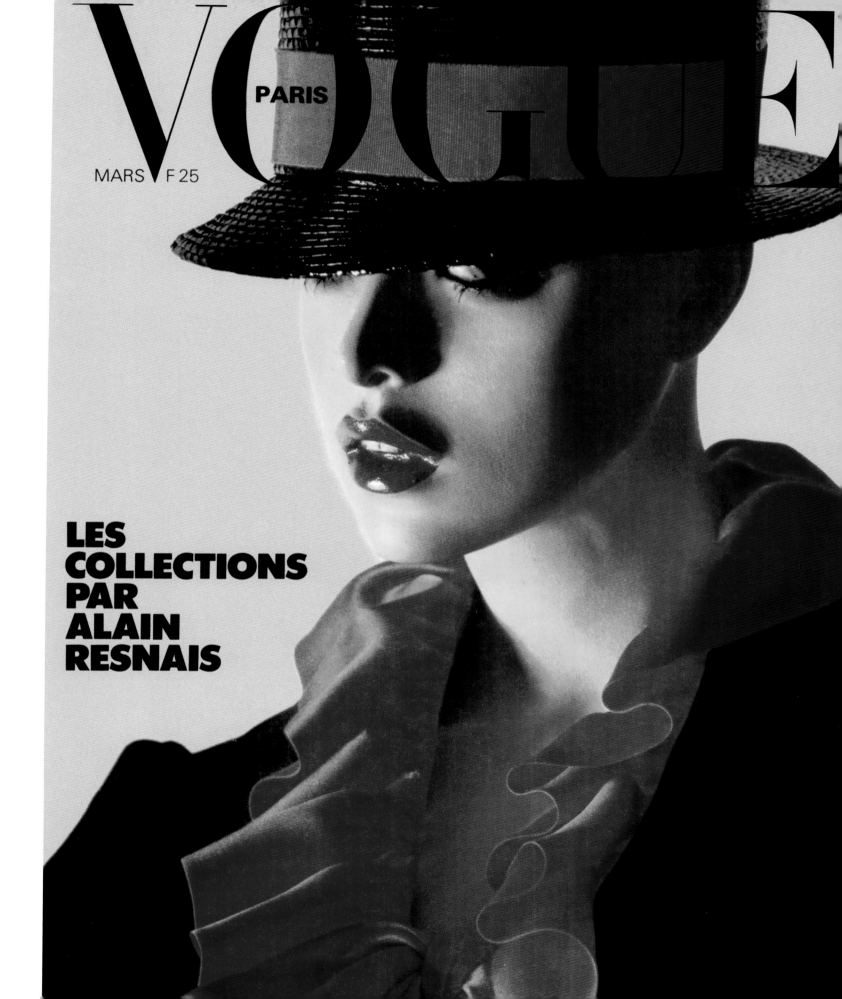

VOGUE

PARIS

MARS ▾ F 25

LES
COLLECTIONS
PAR
ALAIN
RESNAIS

PREVIOUS PAGES
August 2008
Inez van Lamsweerde
& Vinoodh Matadin
Model Daria Werbowy
Couturier Dior

March 1978
Helmut Newton
Couturier Yves Saint Laurent

OPPOSITE
November 2008
Mert Alas & Marcus Piggott
Vanessa Paradis
Couturier Miu Miu

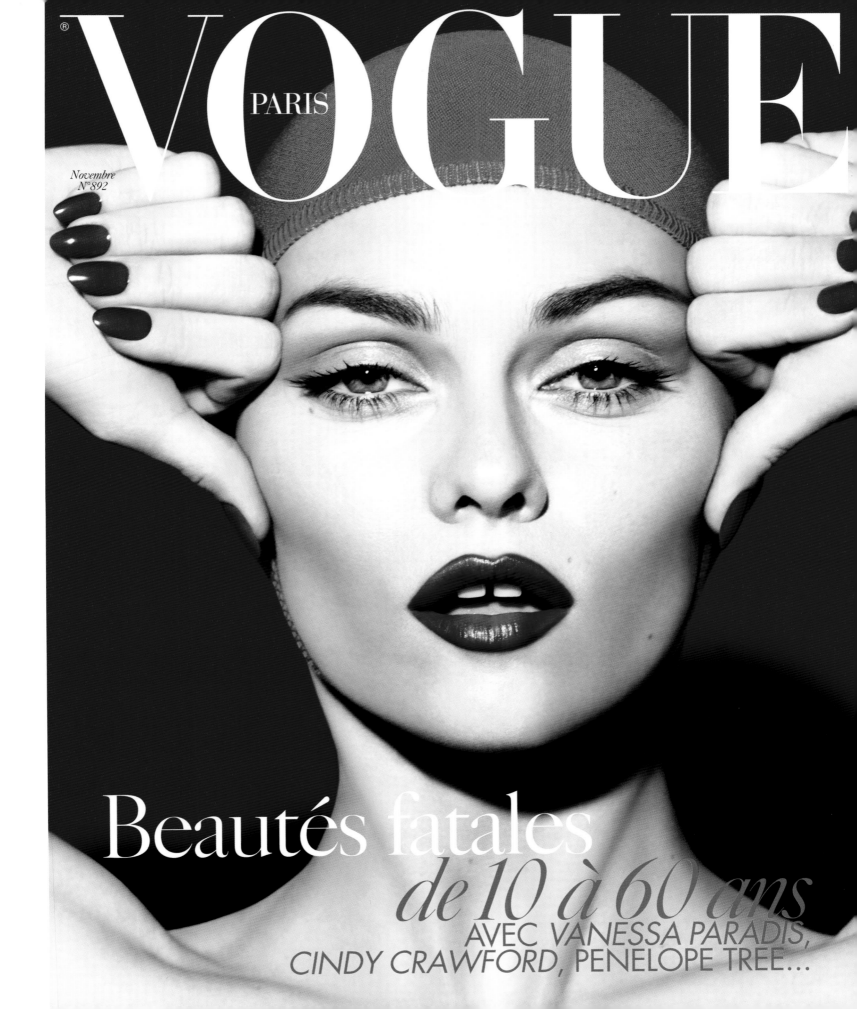

VOGUE
PARIS

Novembre
N° 892

Beautés fatales
de 10 à 60 ans
AVEC VANESSA PARADIS,
CINDY CRAWFORD, PENELOPE TREE…

Bibliography

— *Always in Vogue*, Edna Woolman Chase, Doubleday, 1954.
— *Photographies de mode: 1920–1980*, introduction by Alexander Liberman, Éditions du Fanal, 1980.
— *The Man Who Was Vogue: The Life and Times of Condé Nast*, Caroline Seebohm, Viking, 1982.
— *Les années 20, l'âge des métropoles*, Jean Clair, Gallimard, 1991.
— *Vogue* No. 763, Dec. 1995/Jan. 1996: *Le fabuleux album des 75 ans.*
— *Newhouse: All the Glitter, Power, & Glory of America's Richest Media Empire & the Secretive Man Behind It*, Thomas Maier, Johnson Books, 1997.
— *Mode du siècle*, François Baudot, Assouline, 1999.
— *Lee Miller: A Life*, Carolyn Burke, Knopf, 2005.
— *Magazine Covers*, David Crowley, Mitchell Beazley, 2005.
— *100 Years of Fashion Illustration*, Cally Blackman, Laurence King, 2007.
— *Edward Steichen: In High Fashion – The Condé Nast Years, 1923–1937*, Todd Brandow and William A. Ewing, W. W. Norton & Co., 2008.

Credits

Cover
Newton, Helmut
(© The Helmut Newton Estate /
Maconochie Photography)

Alas, Mert, & Piggott, Marcus
    (© Vogue Paris) pp. 80, 99, 203
Avedon, Richard
    (© The Richard Avedon Foundation)
    p. 195
Bailey, David
    (© Vogue Paris) pp. 47, 56, 166, 187
Benito, Eduardo
    (© Condé Nast Archive) pp. 20, 21, 26,
    27, 28, 31, 141
Breitenmoser
    (© Vogue Paris) p. 55
Chagall, Marc
    (© Vogue Paris) p. 126
Chateau, René
    (© Vogue Paris) p. 156
Clarke, Henry
    (© ADAGP, Paris 2009) pp. 50, 62, 179
Coltellacci, G.
    (© Vogue Paris) pp. 136, 137, 175
Dalí, Salvador
    (© Salvador Dalí, Fondation Gala-
    Salvador Dalí / ADAGP, Paris 2009)
    pp. 122, 123
Demarchelier, Patrick
    (© Vogue Paris) p. 191
Doisneau, Robert
    (© Vogue Paris) pp. 138, 176

Dryden, Helen
    (© Condé Nast Archive) p. 10
Elgort, Arthur
    (© Vogue Paris) p. 92
François, André (Farkas, André, dit)
    (© ADAGP, Paris 2009) p. 188
Halsman, Philippe
    (© Vogue Paris) pp. 107, 123
Hockney, David
    Oil on canvas, 12 1/2 x 9 1/2
    (© David Hockney for French Vogue)
    p. 117
Horst, Horst P.
    (© Condé Nast Archive)
    pp. 37, 39, 87
    (© Vogue Paris) p. 52
Hoyningen-Huene, George
    (© Vogue Paris) p. 38
Kazan, Lionel
    (© Vogue Paris) p. 54
Keogh, Tom
    (© Vogue Paris) p. 196
King, Bill
    (© Vogue Paris) pp. 65, 71
Klein, Steven
    (© Vogue Paris) p. 152
Klein, William
    (© Vogue Paris) pp. 140, 162

This book was published on the occasion of the exhibition 'Vogue Covers 1920-2009'
held from 1 October to 1 November 2009, Champs-Élysées, Paris.

Translated from the French *Vogue Covers 1920-2009* by Ruth Sharman

First published in the United Kingdom in 2009 by
Thames & Hudson Ltd, 181A High Holborn,
London WC1V 7QX
www.thamesandhudson.com

First published in 2009 in hardcover in the United States of America by
Thames & Hudson Inc., 500 Fifth Avenue, New York, New York 10110
thamesandhudsonusa.com

Reprinted in 2011

British Library Cataloguing-in-Publication Data
A catalogue record for this book is available from the British Library

Library of Congress Catalog Card Number 2009932786

ISBN: 978-0-500-51513-6

Printed and bound in Hong Kong